Embryos, Ethics, and Women's Rights
Exploring the New Reproductive Technologies

Embryos, Ethics, and Women's Rights
Exploring the New Reproductive Technologies

Elaine Hoffman Baruch
Amadeo F. D'Adamo, Jr.
Joni Seager
Editors

Embryos, Ethics, and Women's Rights: Exploring the New Reproductive Technologies was simultaneously issued by The Haworth Press, Inc., under the same title, as a special issue of the journal *Women & Health*, Volume 13, Nos. 1/2 1987, Jeanne Stellman, journal editor.

Harrington Park Press
New York • London

ISBN 0-918393-45-0

Published by

Harrington Park Press, Inc., 12 West 32 Street, New York, New York 10001
EUROSPAN/Harrington, 3 Henrietta Street, London WC2E 8LU England

Harrington Park Press, Inc., is a subsidiary of The Haworth Press, Inc., 12 West 32 Street, New York, New York 10001.

Embryos, Ethics, and Women's Rights: Exploring the New Reproductive Technologies was originally published as *Women & Health,* Volume 13, Numbers 1/2 1987.

Cover design by Marshall Andrews

LIBRARY OF CONGRESS
Library of Congress Cataloging-in-Publication Data

Embryos, ethics, and women's rights : exploring the new reproductive technologies / Elaine Hoffman Baruch, Amadeo F. D'Adamo, Jr., Joni Seager, editors.
    p. cm.
    Issued also by: New York : Haworth Press, c1988.
    Has also been published as: Women & health, v. 13, nos. 1/2 1987.
    Rewritten and updated papers presented at two conferences held in New York and Massachusetts in Nov. 1985.
    Bibliography: p.
    ISBN 0-918383-45-0
    1. Human reproduction — Technological innovations — Congresses.
    2. Women's rights — Congresses. 3. Human reproduction — Technological innovations — Moral and ethical aspects — Congresses. 4. Human reproduction — Technological innovations — Social aspects — Congresses. I. Baruch, Elaine Hoffman. II. D'Adamo, Amadeo F. III. Seager, Joni.
    [DNLM: 1. Ethics, Medical — congresses. 2. Fetal Monitoring — congresses. 3. Prenatal Diagnosis — congresses. 4. Reproduction Technics — congresses. 5. Women's Rights — congresses. WQ 205 E535] QP251.E47 1988b
612'.63 — dc19
DNLM/DLC
for Library of Congress   87-38148
                                                      CIP

CONTENTS

ABOUT THE EDITORS

Elaine Hoffman Baruch is Professor of English at York College of the City University of New York, where she teaches a course on literature and biomedical ethics. She is the author of numerous articles on women, literature, and psychoanalysis, the co-editor of *Women in Search of Utopia*, and the co-author of a forthcoming book, *Women Analyze Women: In France, England, and the United States*.

Amadeo F. D'Adamo, Jr. is Professor of Biology at York College of the City University of New York, where he has been Project Director of the Minority Biomedical Research Support Program. He has published extensively in biochemistry, neurobiology, science and ethics.

Joni Seager is the Coordinator of Women's Studies at the Massachusetts Institute of Technology. She is also the Associate Editor for North America for *Women's Studies International Forum*. She has long been active in feminist politics, and especially international feminism. Her recently published book is *Women in the World: An International Atlas*.

Contributors to the Conference

Mary Sue Henifin is an attorney associated with the law firm of Debevoise & Plimpton and Women's Health and the Law Editor for *Women & Health*. As a member of the "Reproductive Laws for the 1990's Project," co-sponsored by the Rutgers University Women's Rights Litigation Clinic and the Institute for Research on Women, she is drafting model state legislation on new reproductive technologies.

YORK COLLEGE OF CUNY CONTRIBUTORS

Elaine Hoffman Baruch is Professor of English at York College of CUNY, where she teaches a course on literature and biomedical ethics. She is the author of numerous articles on women, literature, and psychoanalysis, the co-editor of *Women in Search of Utopia*, and the co-author of a forthcoming book, *Women Analyze Women: In France, England, and the United States*.

Amadeo F. D'Adamo, Jr. is Professor of Biology at York College of CUNY, where he has been Project Director of the Minority Biomedical Research Support Program. He has published extensively in biochemistry and neurobiology as well as on science and ethics.

Alta Charo was Fulbright-Hays Junior Lecturer in American Law at the Université de Paris I (Pantheon-Sorbonne) and was formerly Lecturer-in-Law at the Columbia University School of Law, where she was Associate Director of the Legislative Drafting Research Fund. She is the author of numerous articles on law, science and technology and is currently working in Washington, D.C.

Ruth Hubbard is Professor of Biology at Harvard University and has written many articles and edited several collections, such as *Biological Woman – The Convenient Myth*, *Genes and Gender: Pitfalls in Research on Sex and Gender*, and *Woman's Nature: Rationalizations of Inequality*. Her major professional interests are how questions and answers in science are shaped by the sex, race, and class of scientists and by the social institutions in which they operate, and in the politics of health care, especially as it affects women.

Rev. Ronald D. Lawler is Director of the Institute for Advanced Studies in Catholic Doctrine, St. John's University, and a member of the Pontifical Roman Theological Academy. He is the author of several books, among them, *Philosophical Analysis* and *Catholic Sexual Ethics*.

Betty Jean Lifton is the author of several articles and books, including *Twice Born: Memoirs of an Adopted Daughter*, *Lost and Found: The Adoption Experience*, and *I'm Still Me*, a novel which explores the issues of adoption and the search for identity by a young adult.

Judith Lorber is Professor of Sociology at Brooklyn College and the Graduate Center, CUNY. She is also Director of the Ph.D. Medical Sociology Program of the CUNY Graduate Center and the author of *Women Physicians: Careers, Status, and Power* and numerous articles on women's health issues, patient-staff interaction, and the social construction of gender. Her current research is on the social organization of *in vitro* fertilization, particularly the experiences of clients.

Joseph Anthony Mazzeo retired in 1985 as Avalon Foundation Professor in the Humanities at Columbia University. He published widely in Renaissance Literature, the history of ideas, theory of interpretation and the relations between literature and science. He is currently completing studies in the literature of late antiquity.

Tabitha M. Powledge is editor of *The Scientist*, a new newspaper for scientists, published by the Institute for Scientific Information (Philadelphia). For many years, she was the Director of the Genetics Research Group at the Hastings Center. She was also a senior editor of *Bio/Technology*, the sister journal of *Nature* (London).

John A. Robertson is the Baker and Botts Professor of Law at the University of Texas School of Law, in Austin. He has written extensively on bioethical issues, including the issue of reproductive freedom and is a member of the Ethics Committee of the American Fertility Society.

Barbara Katz Rothman is Professor of Sociology at Baruch College and the Graduate Center of the City University of New York. She is the author of *In Labor*, available in paperback as *Giving Birth*, and *The Tentative Pregnancy: Prenatal Diagnosis And The Future Of Motherhood*.

William Ruddick teaches in both the Philosophy Department and the School of Medicine at New York University. He has written on various topics in medical ethics, including fetal therapy, maternal surrogacy, and parental decisions about treatment of children. He has edited *Philosophers in Medical Centers* and (with Onora O'Neill) *Having Children: Philosophical and Legal Reflections on Parenthood*.

Eleanor Schuker is a Training and Supervising Analyst at the Columbia University Psychoanalytic Center, where she teaches a course on gender and sexuality. She has written on clinical issues relating to women, sexual assault victims, and female creativity. In addition to being in private practice, she is an Attending Psychiatrist at the Columbia University Health Service.

MIT CONTRIBUTORS

Donna Cirasole, a graduate of Wellesley College, is currently studying at the Mount Sinai School of Medicine in New York.

Gena Corea, a journalist, is author of *The Hidden Malpractice: How American Medicine Mistreats Women* and *The Mother Machine: Reproductive Technologies from Artificial Insemination to Artificial Wombs*. Along with Janice Raymond, Renate Klein, Robyn Rowland and Jalna Hanmer, she is co-founder of the Feminist

International Network of Resistance to Reproductive and Genetic Engineering (FINRRAGE).

Patricia M. McShane is Assistant Professor of Obstetrics and Gynecology, Harvard Medical School and Medical Director, IVF Program, Brigham and Women's Hospital.

Rayna Rapp teaches anthropology at the New School for Social Research, helps to edit *Feminist Studies* and *Signs*, and has been active in the reproductive rights movement, and the movement for women's studies for over fifteen years.

Rebecca Sarah is a lay midwife, and the mother of two daughters. She has written about women's health in "Family Journal" and in her regular column in the "Somerville Community News." She also teaches courses in Natural Family Planning and Natural Childbirth.

Marsha Saxton is director of the Project on Women and Disability located at the Massachusetts Office of Handicapped Affairs. She is trainer and activist in disability rights, and co-editor of *With Wings, An Anthology of Literature by and about Women with Disabilities*.

Joni Seager is the Coordinator of Women's Studies at MIT. She is also the Associate Editor for North America for *Women's Studies International Forum*. She has long been active in feminist politics, and especially international feminism. Her recent book is *Women in the World: An International Atlas*.

Thomas A. Shannon is Professor of Social Ethics and Religion in the Department of Humanities at Worcester Polytechnic Institute. Prof. Shannon is the author of several works in Bioethics including *An Introduction to Bioethics, Bioethics: Selected Readings*, and *What Are They Saying About Genetic Engineering*.

Caroline Whitbeck has published widely on questions in the philosophy of science, technology and medicine and feminist philosophy. Since 1978 she has been developing a foundation for the examination of the ethical issues in engineering. She served on the faculties of Yale University, Yale Medical School, the State University of New York and the University of Texas Medical School. She is engaged in research at the MIT Center for Technology, Policy, and Industrial Development, and is Lecturer in the Department of Mechanical Engineering.

Preface

The papers in this collection grew out of two conferences on the new reproductive technologies, one held in New York and the other in Massachusetts. In November 1985, York College of CUNY organized a conference at the CUNY Graduate Center entitled "Embryos, Ethics, and Eugenics: A Brave New World?" For their valuable suggestions, we would like to thank Mariam Chamberlain, Mary Brown Parlee, and Sue Rosenberg Zalk. We would also like to thank the New York Council for the Humanities, the CUNY Academy for the Humanities and Sciences, and York College for their generous support. In April of 1986, the Women's Studies Program at the Massachusetts Institute of Technology convened a conference on "Women and Reproductive Technologies." For their work on this conference, we thank Cynthia Brown, Donna Cirasole, and Ruth Perry. We would particularly like to express our gratitude to the authors in this volume who graciously agreed to rewrite and update their papers for publication.

We call this collection an "exploration" because it represents diverse points of view, bringing together perspectives drawn from the clinical to the personal. Our major concern, however, is to make sure that women and their lives remain visible throughout discussion of these issues. Controversies and battles over reproductive technologies are becoming more heated, and will touch all of our lives. We hope this reader will serve as a resource as we each try to come to terms with the promises and problems of these technologies.

Elaine Hoffman Baruch
Amadeo F. D'Adamo, Jr.
Joni Seager

xvii

Introduction:
Women's Health and
the New Reproductive Technologies

Mary Sue Henifin

This volume, *Embryos, Ethics, and Women's Rights: Exploring the New Reproductive Technologies*, is devoted to new procreative possibilities: *in vitro* fertilization, genetic manipulation of embryos, embryo transfer, surrogacy arrangements, prenatal screening, and the fetus as patient. As Amadeo D'Adamo notes in his opening essay on the scientific issues, the new medical procedures raise a host of ethical, legal, social and psychological concerns. These are explored in the later essays.

Reproduction may now be divided among five different "parents": two genetic parents who contribute sperm and ova for *in vitro* fertilization; the birth mother who accepts the transferred embryo, gestates the fetus, and gives birth; and the social parents who rear the child. These genetic, birth, and social parents may be the same persons or different people. The sperm donor might be married to or unrelated to the genetic, gestational or social mother.[1]

The authors in this volume express fear of an uncertain or gloomy future or guarded optimism as human procreation moves from the bedroom to scientists' laboratories to venture capitalists' fertility clinics. These authors range from historian-of-ideas J. A. Mazzeo, who fears state usurpation of technology for tyrannical ends, to science writer Tabitha Powledge, who thinks the state will have to rescue us from commercial usurpation, to Catholic theologian Rev. Ronald Lawler and philosopher Thomas Shannon, who reject some of these technologies under any conditions. Betty Jean Lifton, a writer on the issues of identity in adoption, fears the psychological consequences of the new technologies on the child, particularly if any secrecy is involved. Psychiatrist Eleanor Schuker, however, believes that the new technologies can relieve the psychological pain of infertility, often without causing damage either to the birth mothers or the children involved. As Elaine Baruch reminds us in her essay, "A Womb of His Own," some feminist writers are among those who have forecast a positive future for new reproductive technologies. Both Shulamith Firestone and Marge Piercy have described utopias where women and baby-making are separated to permit more egalitarian relationships between the sexes. Whether the new reproductive technologies are used to enhance or decrease the autonomy of women will depend on who makes decisions about how they are used. Most feminist critics point out that—to date—it is not women who have controlled the development and use of new reproductive technologies. Caroline Whitbeck and Rebecca Sarah provide the framework for a feminist critique of technology. Gena Corea offers insight into the power relationships, the racism, and the sexism that she sees underlying the social development and applications of reproductive technology.

Because I am writing this introduction in the midst of the public uproar over the trial court's decision in the Baby M case, I am not optimistic about who will control the new reproductive options. Judge Sorkow ruled that the surrogacy contract between Mary Beth Whitehead, Baby M's genetic and birth mother, and William Stern, the baby's genetic father was "a valid and enforceable contract pursuant to the law." The Judge did not rest his opinion solely on contract analysis. He went on to perform the traditional "best interests of the child" test which is the legal standard applied in disputes over child custody. He rejected the argument that emphasis on the best interests of the child will permit "an elite upper economic group of people. . . . to use the lower economic group of women to 'make their babies.'" He believed such an argument to be "insensitive and offensive to the intense drive to procreate naturally and when that is impossible, to use what lawful means are possible to gain a child."

The judicial opinion recognized a right to procreate coitally and grafted onto that right the right to procreate noncoitally: "If it is the reproduction that is protected, then the means of reproduction are also to be protected. The value and interests underlying the creation of family are the same by whatever means obtained. This court holds that the protected means extends to the use of surrogates. . . .''

Judge Sorkow failed to acknowledge that the best interest of the child must also take into account the interests of the birth mother. Denial of the birth mother's interests can only lead to guilt for her child. Baby M will grow up realizing that the court, her father, and adoptive mother all subjected her birth mother to painful and humiliating public scrutiny only to legally terminate her mother's right to maintain a relationship with her.

The Judge in the Baby M case agreed that a state "could regulate, indeed should and must regulate the circumstances under which parties enter into reproductive contracts . . ." but he also held that states "could not ban or refuse to enforce such transactions altogether without compelling reason." He concluded that "refusal to enforce these contracts and prohibition of money payments would constitute an unconstitutional interference with procreative liberty since it would prevent childless couples from obtaining the means with which to have families." This decision is in opposition to the Warnock Commission in England, which has recommended that commercial surrogacy be deemed a criminal offense and that contracts not be enforceable in the courts.

Judge Sorkow's opinion echoes the argument that John Robertson makes for recognition of a constitutionally protected right to procreate by any means available, in his article, "Procreative Liberty, Embryos, and Collaborative Reproduction." The right to procreate is among the individual liberty interests protected by the Constitution. But even if courts extend constitutional protections to new reproductive technologies, state laws burdening such rights can withstand challenge if they are narrowly drawn to protect public health.

What are the long term health effects of permitting women to sell their ova, or their capacity to gestate and give birth? It is a federal crime to permit payment for organs beyond the costs of retrieval.[2] Might we not also decide that it is not in the interest of public health in general, and women's health in particular, to permit payment for sale of ova, or gestation? These questions are addressed in Barbara Katz Rothman's article, "Reproductive Technology and the Commodification of Life." Similarly, R. Alta Charo, in her essay on surrogate mothering, argues that it would be possible to permit surrogacy while avoiding the problems of commercialization by prohibiting the activities of commercial brokers. By recognizing the right to engage in private surrogacy arrangements, while reducing the profit-making incentives which encourage exploitative transactions, the state could protect public health while limiting its interference in private reproductive decisions.

Forbidding the sale of gametes, embryos, and gestation may prevent the worst abuses of the new reproductive technologies. Nevertheless, some of the larger social issues lurking behind the growing use of the new reproductive technologies remain unresolved. As we debate the pros and cons of the new reproductive technologies, we turn our attention away from the basic problems of preventing infertility, providing prenatal care, and finding families for the many children who are warehoused in hospitals, institutions, and group homes. If we truly care about the health of women and children, we need to ask why so much attention is focused on new reproductive technologies, when as a society we have not solved fundamental problems such as allocation of medical care and social services.

Couples who attempt to have a child by means of *in vitro* fertilization — embryo transfer (IVF-ET) generally do so because they are infertile and other medical interventions have failed to help them conceive. Patricia McShane's article, *"In Vitro* Fertilization, GIFT, and Related Technologies,"* describes the IVF process and the IVF client profile. The increasing use of IVF-ET comes at a time when epidemiologists are documenting what appears to be a growing wave of infertility. Suggested causes of this infertility include damage to reproductive organs from sexually-transmitted diseases, prior surgical sterilization, IUD-related pelvic inflammatory disease, DES birth defects, delayed childbearing, and occupational and environmental hazards to male and female reproductive systems.[3]

The growing preoccupation with IVF-ET and other new reproductive technologies diverts attention from primary prevention of infertility. This is particularly harmful to poor and minority communities, which have little access to medical care and experience high rates of infertility.[4] Members of these communities do not have the $30,000 to $50,000 it usually costs for the repeated tries it often takes to have a baby by means of IVF-ET, if you are one of the "lucky" couples.[5] The majority of couples attempting to achieve a baby through IVF-ET will not be successful. In 1985, Gena Corea conducted a survey with the help of the *Medical Tribune*. Fifty percent of the IVF-ET clinics responding to the survey had never sent a woman home with a baby. The high cost of IVF-ET and the few live births make the prevention of infertility a more practical solution.

New reproductive technologies permit parents to have a genetic link with their children. But by doing so, they decrease the number of potential adoptive and foster parents. Approximately 36,000 black children in the United States await adoption.[6] In New York City, abandoned babies live in hospital cribs and take their first steps while holding a nurse's hand.[7] We emphasize genetic parenthood but we turn away from the plight of children in need of parents, languishing in institutions. Anthropological evidence, contrary to commonly held assumptions of sociobiologists, suggests that the desire to have children that are genetically-related is not biologically determined but rather culturally constructed.[8]

The new reproductive technologies fuel the desire for genetically-related children and encourage attempts to achieve genetic parenthood at whatever the costs. Yet these technologies provide no answers for children who are in need of social parenting.

New reproductive technologies in the form of prenatal screening similarly fail to address the major causes of infant illness and disability. Prenatal screening permits diagnosis of genetic defects. Therapeutic abortion is the usual "treatment" offered. Marsha Saxton and Rayna Rapp discuss the impact of prenatal screening and discriminatory attitudes about disability. In "Eugenics: New Tools, Old Ideas," Ruth Hubbard evaluates the potential for abuse that prenatal screening affords. As Ruth Hubbard also explains, if we, as a society, are concerned about the health of babies, we should put greater resources into services for women and prenatal care. Low birth weight and prematurity are the major causes of infant illness and death, and these conditions are associated with poverty and lack of access to prenatal care, not with genetic conditions.

This volume raises many questions. Will the attention and monies focused on the new reproductive technologies transfer resources from infertility prevention, prenatal care, and adoption? Will procreation become another technology purchased in the marketplace with "designer" sperm, ova, and embryos offered for sale? Will private agencies arrange, for a fee, the gestation of specially-engineered embryos in the wombs of surrogates? If states move to regulate such practices, will it encourage widespread governmental interference in reproductive choice?

The answers to these questions are not inherent in the new technologies. As sociologist Judith Lorber details, in "*In Vitro* Fertilization and Gender Politics," they will be revealed through the attitudes and actions of those who make decisions about how the procedures will be used. Whereas Lorber documents that men are too often the dominant partner in reproductive decisions, philosopher William Ruddick, in "A Short Answer to 'Who Decides?'" argues that "women, and only women, should make decisions about their own childbearing." As we debate the future of the new reproductive technologies, women must continue trying to define what is best for women, and work to achieve those goals. Whether we look at the history of DES, IUDs or occupational and environmental hazards, it has been illustrated over and over again that abdication of responsibility for public health to the marketplace has had a dismal history of failure.

NOTES

1. A. Capron diagrams the many permutations that may exist among the genetic, birth and social parents in his article, "The New Reproductive Possibilities: Seeking a Moral Basis for Concerted Action in a Pluralistic Society," *Law, Medicine & Health Care* 12 (1984), 192, 194.

2. The federal law that prohibits the sale of organs is codified at 42 U.S.C.A. Sec. 274e (West 1987 Supp.).

3. *See* Aral & Cates, "The Increasing Concern with Infertility," *Journal of the American Medical Association* 250 (1983), 2327; L. Andrews, *New Conceptions: A Consumer's Guide to the Newest Infertility Treatments* (1984).

4. *Ibid.*

5. *See* J. Hollinger, "From Coitus to Commerce: Legal and Social Consequences of Noncoital Reproduction," *Journal of Law Reform* 18 (1985) 865, 872.

6. *N. Y. Times*, April 2, 1987 at A-12.

7. *N. Y. Times*, "A System Overloaded: The Foster Care Crisis," March 15, 1987 at 1.

8. Hollinger, supra note 5 at 874-75. Gena Corea argues this persuasively in her article in this volume.

REFERENCES

Hughes, D., Johnson, K., Rosenbaum, S., Simons, J., and Butler, B. 1987. *The Health of America's Children*, Washington, DC: The Children's Defense Fund.

Milunsky, A. and Annas, G., (eds.) 1985. *Genetics and the Law III*, New York: Plenum Press.

United Kingdom, Department of Health and Social Security. 1984. *Report of the Committee of Inquiry into Human Fertilization and Embryology* (Chairman, Mary Warnock), London: Her Majesty's Stationery Office.

Reproductive Technologies: The Two Sides of the Glass Jar

Amadeo F. D'Adamo, Jr.

SUMMARY. From our knowledge of fertilization and implantation, new methods of reproduction have been developed. These new reproductive technologies make possible new parenting arrangements, resetting the biological clock for women, selecting the timing of birth, sex and number of children, pre-implantation diagnosis and gene replacement. The new ways of making babies present us with a myriad of ethical, legal, social and psychological concerns.

Scientific information changes our perceptions in at least two ways: it leads to an increased understanding of the processes of the universe however we define that universe, whether as our physical universe or the fertilized ovum, and, through technical application of the knowledge gained, it leads to an increased ability to utilize and direct these processes.

Such is the case in human reproduction. We have gone from such misconceptions as Harvey's conclusion in the 1650s that embryos were secreted from the fluids of the uterus under the influence of seminal "effluvium," to an understanding not only of fertilization, implantation and development but also to the application of this knowledge in new methods of reproduction (Short 1977). As a result of using this scientific information, reproductive technology has expanded from artificial insemination by either husband or donor to oocyte collection and *in vitro* fertilization, where sperm and

9

oocyte interact in a glass container (termed *in vitro* fertilization or IVF), followed by embryo transfer (ET) to a physiologically receptive uterus.

Having removed the early steps of reproduction from the natural setting of a woman's body, we have increased our ability to aid infertile couples, and to deliver "state-of-the-art babies." We now confront the myriad legal, economic, ethical and personal aspects of those developments.

In order to discuss these new ways of making babies, some of the principles and terminology involved in the initiation of pregnancy by a coital act will be useful.

THE PHYSIOLOGY OF REPRODUCTION

All the approximately 2,000,000 cells which can mature into potential eggs or ova are already present in the ovaries at birth. The complete maturation of these oocytes requires hormonal signals and two cell divisions over a time sequence; generally only one such maturation will occur in a monthly cycle, all other cells remaining in the resting state. The initial steps in the maturation process occur in regions of the ovary called follicles which become fluid filled, expand to almost one inch in size, and bulge out of the surface of the ovary (see Fig. 1). This fluid, when released by the rupture of the follicle, aids in propelling the maturing oocyte and associated cells towards the Fallopian or uterine tubes. Ultrasound technology takes advantage of this bulging to localize developed oocytes for collection.

What is released from the ovary to the Fallopian tubes in response to a hormonal signal is technically not an ovum but a secondary oocyte — a cell surrounded by a thick, clear membrane or envelope, the zona pellucida and a cluster of other cells (see secondary oocyte — Fig. 2). The second maturation division to an ovum with the correct amount of genetic material will be completed when a spermatozoon penetrates the zona pellucida of the secondary oocyte.

As they are released in ejaculation, sperm do not have the capacity to penetrate this outer cluster of cells and the zona pellucida.

THE OVARY

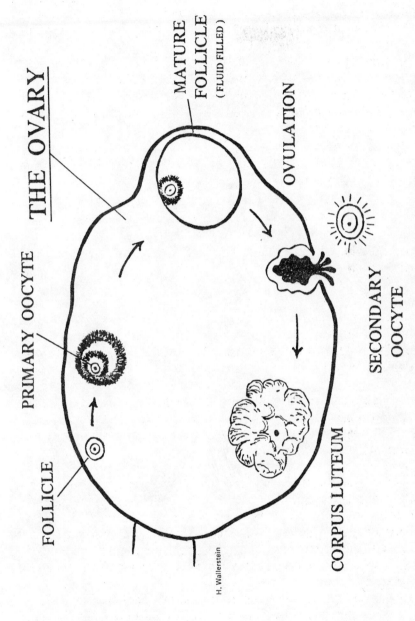

FOLLICLE

PRIMARY OOCYTE

MATURE FOLLICLE (FLUID FILLED)

OVULATION

SECONDARY OOCYTE

CORPUS LUTEUM

H. Wallerstein

FIGURE 1. The development of an ovum.[1] Note the bulging out of the mature follicle from the surface of the ovary.

11

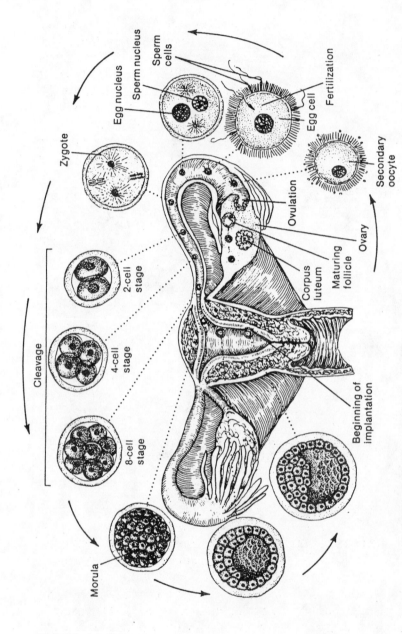

FIGURE 2. Stages in ovulation, fertilization, and implantation. (From Hole, John W., Jr., *Human Anatomy and Physiology*, 4th ed. © 1978, 1981, 1984, 1987 Wm. C. Brown Publishers, Dubuque, Iowa. All Rights Reserved. Reprinted by permission.)

12

They are "capacitated" by substances in the female reproductive system as they travel from the vagina through the uterus to the Fallopian tubes where fertilization actually takes place. (Some forms of male infertility may be a result of difficulties in capacitation.) If fertilization of the secondary oocyte does not occur, then menstruation, a sloughing off of the thickened uterine wall which has been hormonally prepared for a potential pregnancy, will ensue.

If, on the other hand, fertilization does occur, then some important events follow in the Fallopian tubes over the next several days (Fig. 2 – zygote through morula stage):

1. The maternal and paternal chromosomal material mix and the cell, now called a zygote, prepares for a series of cell divisions.

2. The first cell division produces two blastomeres (Fig. 2 – the two cell stage), each of which is not only genetically equivalent but identical in many ways. At this stage, the two blastomeres may separate and identical twins would result. This ability to separate the blastomeres and still develop a complete individual will be discussed later as one aspect of the new reproductive technologies.

3. Within a few days after fertilization, the ball of dividing cells has traveled through the Fallopian tubes and enters the uterine cavity (Fig. 2 – the morula).

The developing cell mass floats free in the uterine cavity and may be recovered by lavage or repeated washing of the uterus. This property has been used as one method of embryo transfer. By day 6, however, the cell mass hatches from the zona pellucida and begins to embed in the uterine wall, establishing the maternal-fetal bond (Fig. 2 – the beginning of implantation). Now other important processes occur, notably:

1. The development of the extra-embryonic membranes including the amnion, which encases the developing fetus in the protecting amniotic fluid. Penetration of this amniotic membrane with a needle to collect fluid containing cells of the fetus is the basis of the diagnostic procedure called amniocentesis.

2. Differentiation into various tissues and organs begins. By day 16 after fertilization the primitive streak which sets the cranial-anal axis appears. (This primitive streak stage will be referred

to in the discussion on the ethics of research on embryos.) By day 18, the central nervous system begins to develop and by week 9 the fetus responds sluggishly to touch.

NONCOITAL FERTILIZATION

This was the sequence of human reproduction until Steptoe and Edwards (1978) of Great Britain delivered Louise Brown, who was conceived using the techniques of *in vitro* fertilization and embryo transfer. They were not, however, the first to use reproductive technology to expand the bounds of traditional coital reproduction. In the late nineteenth century, Walter Heape (1890) had already demonstrated that embryo donation from one female to another physiologically receptive female was possible. In Heape's experiment, two pre-implantation embryos were retrieved by flushing the oviducts of a newly-mated Angora doe rabbit and were transferred to the oviducts of a newly-mated Belgian hare. Of the litter of six which resulted, two were Angora rabbits. In effect, the Belgian hare was the gestational mother—but not the genetic mother of the rabbits.

Combinations of different techniques make it possible for a child to have up to five parents: (1) the sperm donor, who may or may not be the nurturing or social father, (2) the "surrogate mother," who is the genetic mother who has been artificially inseminated but has no intention of rearing the child herself, (3) the gestational mother, who has been implanted with an embryo to which she has made no genetic contribution, but which she carries to term for herself or for others, (4) the nurturing or social mother, who rears the child but has made no genetic contribution to it, (5) the nurturing or social father (Baruch and D'Adamo 1985). (In England, the term *surrogate mother* is used for both 2 and 3.)

The procedure now generally used for *in vitro* fertilization and embryo transfer is not that initially developed by Steptoe and Edwards but a modification introduced by Trounson and his co-workers in Australia, which encompasses five steps (see McBain and Trounson 1984; Mohr and Trounson 1984; Trounson et al. 1981).

1. A woman is treated between day 5 and 9 after menstruation starts with the drug Clomiphene citrate to initiate the maturation of the oocytes. This hyperstimulates the ovary so that several follicles mature rather than just one as in the usual cycle. During the treatment she is given blood tests and examined by ultrasound to determine whether oocytes are properly developing. As they near maturity, another hormone is given to aid release. Of course, the oocytes should not be so mature that they spontaneously leave the ovary and thus cannot be retrieved.

2. At this point, the woman is subjected to general anaesthesia followed by surgery and a laparoscopy. (The laparoscope is a long, thin telescopic instrument which enables the surgeon to see those oocytes that have properly matured.)

3. The mature oocytes are removed by gentle suction or aspiration through a specially constructed hollow needle. A retrieval success rate of 90% is common. More recently, ultrasound guided retrieval with a success rate of 50% has been developed. While the retrieval rate is lower, the ultrasound procedure is less invasive: it requires only a local anaesthetic which results in less trauma to the woman and is much less expensive. These super-ovulation techniques make it possible to retrieve several mature secondary oocytes at one time, thus allowing the production of more embryos than are required for one implantation cycle. The availability of excess embryos makes possible embryo research, embryo selection, embryo storage by freezing and embryo donation. These alternatives to immediate implantation are responsible for many of the ethical, psychological, social and legal concerns that this technology presents.

4. In the meantime, the man masturbates to collect sperm. However, there are now available special condoms so that sperm may be obtained in the more traditional coital act. The sperm obtained are capacitated during the preparation technique for *in vitro* fertilization.

5. A secondary oocyte is placed in an incubation medium in a glass dish. Sperm are then added. (Since many fewer sperm are required than in a coital act, *in vitro* fertilization may be effective in overcoming some types of male infertility.) Once fertilized and al-

lowed to proceed through a few cell divisions, the embryo is transferred to the uterus of a physiologically receptive woman where it
may implant. (The generalized procedure is shown in Fig. 3.)

SUCCESS RATE AND COSTS

The success rate in these procedures varies greatly from institution to institution. In the best programs approximately 75% of the
oocytes retrieved are found, on microscopic examination, to have
been successfully fertilized. Workers in the Monash University
clinic in Australia have found a 13% rate of pregnancy when only
one embryo is transferred which increases to 35% if three are transferred (McBain and Trounson 1984). Obviously, the transfer of
more than one embryo at a time increases the potential for multiple
births – the world's first quadruple birth from these techniques occurred in Australia in 1984. Increasing the number of transfer attempts also increases the pregnancy rate on a proportional basis.
When these techniques were first devised, each transfer attempt required a laparoscopy and aspiration to obtain oocytes. These repeated procedures were not only expensive but traumatic, since
each new attempt required a general anesthesia of the woman. A
way around this problem has been found. Several oocytes are retrieved during a laparoscopy, then fertilized and developed to the
eight cell stage. These are frozen in liquid nitrogen, and stored –
then if needed, thawed and transferred sequentially if the previous
attempt did not result in a live birth.

Only about 10% of the total *in vitro* fertilization and embryo
transfer attempts per cycle result in a live birth. The cost of this
technology is quite high: it has been estimated that the cost of the
entire procedure is approximately $5,500 for the first attempt
(Grobstein et al. 1983; Bellina and Wilson 1985). Once the preliminary testing is done, subsequent attempts are less expensive. Given
that there is a 10% chance of having a live birth for each attempt,
one can see that a couple may spend up to $30,000 to have a 50%
chance of having a child. The total potential expenditures on the
new reproductive technologies should not be underestimated. In the

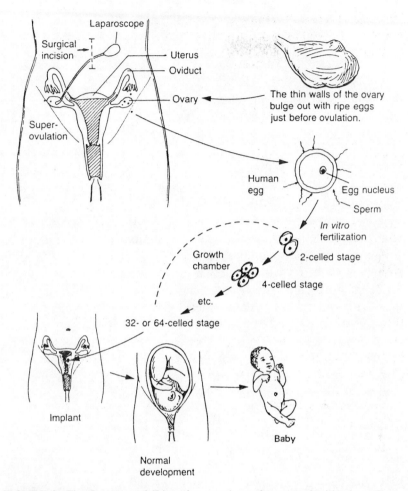

FIGURE 3. The Steptoe and Edwards procedure of *in vitro* fertilization. (From Kieffer, *Bioethics: A Textbook of Issues,* © 1979 The Benjamin/Cummings Publishing Co., reprinted with permission.)[3]

United States approximately one out of eight couples can be classified as infertile. It has been estimated that 70,000 American women a year will seek to use these procedures (Center for Disease Control 1982, Blank 1985).

OTHER TECHNIQUES

Other types of techniques have been developed to treat infertility. One recent innovation is the GIFT method or Gametic Intra-Fallopian Transfer. In this method, secondary oocytes obtained by laparoscopy or ultrasound procedures are mixed with sperm and transferred back into the Fallopian tubes. Since this approach closely simulates the traditional coital method it is hoped that a success rate greater than 10% live births per treatment will be achieved. The researchers involved plan world-wide trials for 500 women in the near future (Asch et al. 1984).

A live human birth has occurred using a modification of the lavage method mentioned earlier which was first used with rabbits by Walter Heape one hundred years ago. The husband of an infertile woman who had an intact uterus but could not produce oocytes impregnated a surrogate by artificial insemination. The cycles of the two women were synchronized by hormonal treatment of the infertile woman. Before implantation occurred, the embryo was washed out of the uterus of the surrogate donor and successfully transferred to the infertile recipient. Thus, the infertile woman became the gestational mother and the nurturing mother but since the oocyte fertilized was not hers, she is not the genetic mother of the child she gave birth to (Bustello et al. 1984).

In this respect, it should be pointed out that the gestational mother need not be, in fact, of the same species as the genetic mother. A zebra was recently born from a zebra embryo transferred to the uterus of a mare who became the gestational mother (see Fig. 4). It is likely, although I find it ethically and aesthetically repugnant that such trans-species gestations can occur in which other primates carry human fetuses.

In vitro fertilization was initially developed to assist women with defective or blocked Fallopian tubes to achieve a pregnancy. Microsurgical techniques are now available to obtain sperm from the testes in cases where the male is unable to ejaculate normally or is unable to generate the large numbers needed for successful reproduction.

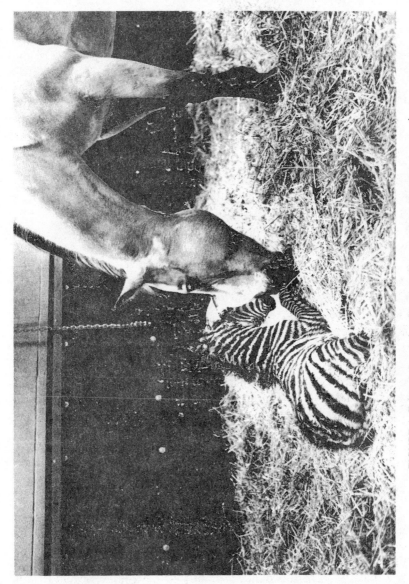

FIGURE 4. *Zebra and gestational mother.* Photograph by Paul Schuhmann. 4

IMPLICATIONS OF THE NEW TECHNOLOGIES

These new technologies allow the initial stages of pregnancy to occur in a glass jar. Thus not only do they enable a child to have up to five parents, but they make possible a change in the mechanism and timing of reproduction, as well as certain kinds of testing and intervention. The remainder of this paper will discuss what the implications of these procedures are from a scientific viewpoint. Ethical, legal, social and psychological ramifications are dealt with in other papers in this book.

Since 1983, it has been possible to freeze human embryos in liquid nitrogen and, after thawing, implant them months and perhaps years after fertilization. Several children have since been born using this technique of cryostorage (Trounson and Mohr 1983; Trounson 1986). Frozen oocyte technology is a very recent development; in the summer of 1986 the first children were born in Australia from frozen oocytes which were thawed after being frozen for only a few minutes. The thawed oocytes were then fertilized and transferred, resulting in a successful pregnancy. Dr. Christopher Chen who developed this technique reports that there is now an ongoing pregnancy from an oocyte that had been frozen for several months before thawing (personal communication by telephone, August 6, 1986). He suggests that in the near future there will be oocyte banks available, organized in a fashion similar to sperm banks. Unlike semen collection, however, retrieving oocytes requires hormonal and surgical intervention which may have some risks and discomfort for the woman.

Limits on the length of time that the tissue can remain in cryostorage have been recommended. In Australia, where many of these techniques have been developed, guidelines of the National Health and Medical Research Council limits cryostorage to 10 years. Putting aside the biological considerations, unlimited cryostorage and then implantation particularly across generational intervals raises major concerns (Trounson 1986).

Yet, even within this time limit, one possibility raised by these new methods of reproduction is the resetting of the biological clock for women so that the child-bearing years may be extended. Generally women fear delaying having children until the age of forty or beyond in ways that men do not. Although paternal aging is implicated in a few chromosomal disorders, its role in most birth abnormalities is not definite. By contrast, the reproductive years for a woman are more limited. The total number of ova are present at birth, and these seem to be subject to aging. Fetal chromosomal disorders increase two- to three-fold when mothers are over 40 as compared with those just a few years younger. In children born to mothers who are forty-five years old there are an average of 53 chromosomal abnormalities per 1,000 births in contrast to 2 when the mother is age twenty-five at the birth of the child (Milunsky, 1979).

Now that methods for the freezing and thawing of human oocytes and embryos are available, the time interval between oocyte retrieval and implantation may be extended for months and perhaps years allowing a woman to choose the time of pregnancy and at the same time bypass the aging problem. The difference between the age of the uterus and that of the embryo appears not to be critical. Recently a woman in her forties, with a long history of infertility, gave birth to a normal infant after embryo transfer, using an oocyte from a thirty-two year old donor (Rosenwaks, Veeck and Liu 1986). Indeed, a 48-year-old grandmother has successfully carried three fetuses from her own daughter's oocytes; she is the gestational mother of children who are genetically her grandchildren (Battersby 1987:1). Whether the uterus of a post-menopausal woman is still physiologically functional and capable of sustaining a pregnancy is not known at the present time.

Some women over forty may not wish to carry the fetus, although they want to be the genetic mothers. The solution to this problem through the use of gestational mothers has already been mentioned. Such implantation may be desirable under other circumstances, for example, if the uterine environment of the genetic mother is harmful to fetal development, either because of her own genetic makeup, or her exposure to toxic substances at the workplace, or for reasons of her own health.

When these techniques are used to change the biological clock, stored frozen oocytes will probably be the most frequent choice. Stored embryos, in contrast to stored oocytes, lock a woman into reproduction with the particular male whose sperm fertilized the oocyte but who may no longer be present years later because of divorce or death.

These freezing techniques lead to a number of problems. Who will have custody of frozen embryos in the event of a couple's divorce? Should parents have access to the frozen oocytes or embryos of a daughter who has died? If it is the male partner who has died and the woman decides against implantation, what are the rights of *his* parents to the frozen embryos or his frozen sperm? Is there a right to be a grandparent, and does this right extend to obtaining sperm (a simple process) or ova (an invasive and potentially harmful procedure) from a sick or dying child? What are the legal and ethical implications if fertilization or implantation is done after one or both of the biological parents have died (Baruch and D'Adamo 1985)?

In addition to resetting the biological clock by extending the childbearing years, the new reproductive technology may telescope the time required to have several children. It may be possible for a woman who wants a family of two or three children to have them at the same time rather than over several years. Super-ovulation procedures, now used to counter some forms of infertility, frequently result in multiple births. However, a safer and more controlled method may be through *in vitro* fertilization and embryo transfer.

This technology may also be used to have identical twins by separating the blastomeres at the two cell or four cell stage. In theory, the technique is as simple as using a looped hair to separate the cells, each one of which will develop individually (see Fig. 5). A similar method was used more than a generation ago with other species (Horstadius and Wolsky 1936). Separation of the blastomeres at an early stage also occurs naturally, leading to identical twins. Embryo-splitting methods to clone precise replicas of cattle and other livestock have already been developed (Schneider 1987).

PRE-IMPLANTATION DIAGNOSIS
AND ITS IMPLICATIONS

The capability of separating the blastomeres before implantation will also change the mechanism and timing of prenatal diagnosis. Present prenatal diagnostic techniques other than ultra-sound re-

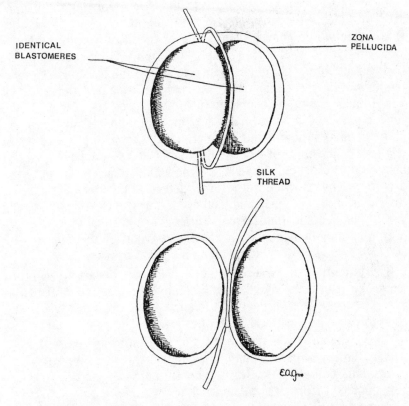

FIGURE 5. Embryo-splitting for induced twinning or pre-implantation diagnosis. [5]

quire invasive procedures; for these, the pregnancy must be well beyond the initial stage. Amniocentesis, one of the most common diagnostic tools for chromosomal examination, also reveals the sex of the fetus. It cannot be done until about the 16th week of pregnancy and a diagnosis may not be available until 22 weeks of gestation. Chorionic villi sampling, which removes cells from the placenta for examination after eight weeks of pregnancy, is still in the experimental stage. At the very least, the woman has to go through the psychological stress of waiting for test results while carrying the fetus.

In contrast, blastomere separation and "pre-implantation diagnosis" provides the opportunity to study—and select—embryos before the actual pregnancy occurs. This capability for pre-implantation diagnosis will bring important benefits. Separating the undifferentiated blastomeres will provide a sample of cells for examination; the remaining cells, encased in a zona pellucida, will be kept frozen. Using molecular probes, the test cells can be examined for the presence of abnormal genes, potential genetic diseases and chromosomal structure and number. Thus, for example, one could test for the presence of sickle cell anemia or Tay-Sachs disease, or any known biochemical defect. One could test for Down Syndrome, or any known chromosomal defect. If this pre-implantation diagnosis shows no measurable abnormalities, then the stored cells can be thawed and transferred. Women would be able to use this pre-implantation diagnosis, performed outside of the time of the actual pregnancy, to decide which embryo to bring to term.

The potential for pre-implantation diagnosis does lead to problems. While parents have the right to know the negative information available from pre-implantation diagnosis, should they have the right to use it as a method of sex pre-selection?

The desire to predetermine the sex of a child has existed from ancient times. Aristotle maintained that boys were conceived by having intercourse in the North wind and girls in the South wind. Hippocrates' theory of sex determination was based on a sexist conception of body geography: sperm for males, he asserted, were located in the right testicle (on the just and good side of the body); that for girls in the left (the devious side). To have a boy, he recommended that a man tie off his left testicle and have the woman lie on her right side after intercourse, this being the side of the uterus for male implantation. In more recent times, attempts to control the sex of a child have included techniques for the separation of X bearing sperm (which produce a girl) from Y bearing ones (which produce a boy). Perhaps the most recent method suggested is that of monoclonal antibodies as a sex selective spermicide used in a vaginal foam or jelly during natural intercourse. These antibodies, either anti X or anti Y, would destroy the sperm leading to the unwanted sex, presenting the oocyte with only those of the desired sex (Rothberg 1986).

Amniocentesis is now widely used in China and India to determine the sex of the fetus. Because the pressure for one-child families is strong in China, and because males are preferred in both countries, female fetuses are frequently aborted (Davin 1985). Thus reproductive technology is used for femicide. There appears to be an increasing use of amniocentesis in this country, too, for sex selection (Mittenthal 1984). Parents generally want to have boys first (Westoff and Rindfuss 1974). The advanced pre-implantation diagnosis, which enables the sex to be chosen before the actual pregnancy, could institutionalize this bias. The resulting older brother/younger sister pattern would, no doubt, increase male dominance. Such technology, if applied, might also change the sex ratio, with unforeseen results for the future.

Other pre-implantation or prenatal diagnostic tests and procedures raise new questions. When molecular probes become available to test embryos for growth hormone and other developmental factors, would parents have the right to choose the embryo which will develop into the tallest male or shortest female to fit their stereotypes of masculinity and femininity? If the embryos on hand do not meet the genetic specification of the parents, what are the ethical considerations in disposing of that group of embryos and producing another set? (For a discussion of the theory and technique of genetic probes, see Miller 1984.)

The availability of separated blastomeres and pre-implantation of diagnosis may also ultimately make possible gene replacement therapy in which an abnormal gene is removed from a blastomere and by gene splicing replaced with a normal gene. Thus the germ cells of this individual, when produced years later, will not have the abnormal genes. Yet the same technique of replacement therapy could be used by parents to substitute for normal genes in order to have, for example, a blue-eyed person by substituting for the genetic information which would have led to a brown-eyed person, or vice-versa. In this way, individual preferences in the use of these new technologies in the search for the perfect child could affect the gene pool of the entire human race.

It is also difficult to assess the long term end results, dangers as well as benefits, of other types of the new reproductive technology. For example, microinjection techniques, which involve the injection of genetic material into an oocyte through a very thin, hollow needle, might be used in aiding infertile men whose sperm cannot penetrate the zona pellucida. In this case, the entire genetic material would be injected into the oocyte and one would anticipate a normal pregnancy and development. If, however, only fragments of the genetic material are transferred, as in the case of injecting only that portion of genetic material which regulates growth hormone, all of the effects on the individual may not be known for years. When such a fusion gene experiment was performed with mice, there was in fact a 50% increase in size (Hammer et al. 1984). However, when the animals reached reproductive age, it was found that only one in ten females were fertile whereas male fertility increased. What this illustrates is that development is a lifetime process. In the continuum from fertilization through 70 or 80 years, problems may arise which were not anticipated in the initial genetic engineering procedure.

While these gene replacement therapies and microinjection procedures refer to individual choices, perhaps the greatest fear of the widespread development of reproductive engineering is that a totalitarian government might manipulate the production of germ cells and embryos and a presetting of the genetic program for its own use. Using pre-implantation diagnosis, a government might dictate that each blastocyst be tested for resistance to a specific group of carcinogens, pesticides, or to radiation so that implantation and development would provide workers for the industrial and agricultural establishment or the nuclear industry. Clearly, physical types favored by autocratic regimes, such as the Nazi model of the tall, blue-eyed Aryan, would now be achievable.

EMBRYONIC TISSUE
AND BIOLOGICAL PERSONHOOD

It is in precisely this increase in the potential to abuse human bodies that the greatest ethical, legal and psychological concerns about the new reproductive technology arise. Should human embryonic tissue be made available for the industrial production of important medicinal products such as insulin? Should embryos be developed beyond the primitive streak stage, which just precedes the development of the nervous system, solely for the purpose of providing siblings with replacement parts?

The limited availability of organs such as kidneys or heart for transplants is a serious and growing problem. It is possible to replace the genetic material in an ovum at the pronuclei stage, which occurs immediately after fertilization, with the genetic material of a specific male or female. Thus one individual could provide both sets of genetic information and the developing fetus would have its genetic complement from only one person. (This is not the same as the cloning procedure suggested by David Rorvik in *In His Image: The Cloning of a Man*.) If this person needs a tissue transplant, is it ethical to develop a fetus to a specific point, abort it and remove the tissue needed?

From a spiritual perspective, the question of when a unique human soul is infused in a cell or groups of cells is an important one. Scientific discoveries and principles cannot answer this question. Yet central to the answer is understanding when and how unique biological personhood occurs. Twinning from one set of blastomeres reveals that there is the potential for a group of cells to develop into more than one individual. Once blastomeres in Petri dishes were available, other kinds of information on this issue could be obtained. For example, it is possible to combine blastomeres from strains of white coated mice and black coated mice and obtain individuals, called chimeras, who have black and white stripes (Fig. 6). These are each distinct individuals having the genetic material of four parents and two sets of cells which are genetically different (Mintz 1962; Tarkowski 1964). If this procedure were to be carried out with human blastomeres, would what was presumably two souls now be merged—or would a new third one be developed? Clearly, scientific research using reproductive technology shows that biological personhood may be more complex than previously assumed.

Many critics of the new reproductive technologies maintain that these techniques manufacture babies. Children born through the use of these technologies are in no way put together through a quality control process like an automobile or a combining of bits and pieces

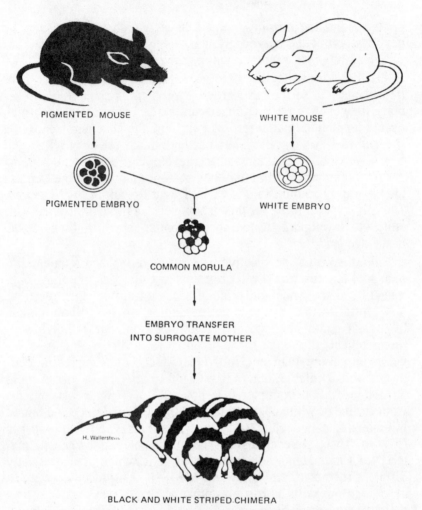

PIGMENTED MOUSE

WHITE MOUSE

PIGMENTED EMBRYO

WHITE EMBRYO

COMMON MORULA

EMBRYO TRANSFER
INTO SURROGATE MOTHER

H. Wallerstein

BLACK AND WHITE STRIPED CHIMERA

FIGURE 6. Mouse Aggregation Chimeras.[6]

like Frankenstein's monster.[6] Which follicles will mature, which oocytes will be fertilized and by which sperm is no more controllable or predictable in this process than in the traditional coital act. These children will be as biologically and personally unique as in traditional reproduction and will surprise, delight and vex their parents as children always have since humans began to procreate.

NOTES

Some of this material appears in E. H. Baruch and A. F. D'Adamo, Jr. 1985. "Resetting the Biological Clock." *Dissent* Summer Issue: 273-276.

1. Fig. 1 and 6 drawn by Harold Wallerstein.

2. Fig. 2 From J. W. Hole, Jr. 1978 *Human Anatomy and Physiology* 3d ed. (c) 1978, 1981, 1984, 1987, p. 837. Wm. C. Brown Publishers, Dubuque, Iowa.

3. Fig. 3 From G. H. Kieffer. 1979. *Bioethics: A Textbook of Issues* Fig. 3 and 4. The Benjamin/Cummings Publishing Co. Menlo Park, CA.

4. Photograph courtesy of Paul Schuhmann, *The Courier Journal* and *The Louisville Times*. The embryo transfer procedure was performed by W. R. Foster, D.V.M. and S. D. Bennett, D.V.M. at the Louisville Zoo.

5. Fig. 5 drawn by Erica A. Gross.

6. The use of an artificial uterus to carry the embryo to term is theoretically possible. This or trans-species gestation would constitute manufacturing babies.

REFERENCES

Asch, R. H. et al. (1984). "Pregnancy After Translaparoscopic Gamete Intrafallopian Transfer." *Lancet* 1034 (Letter to the Editor).

Baruch, E. H. and A. F. D'Adamo, Jr. 1985. "Resetting the Biological Clock." *Dissent*, Summer Issue: 273-76.

Battersby, J. D. 1987. "Woman is Carrying Her Daughter's Babies." *The New York Times*, April 9:1.

Bellina, J. and J. Wilson. 1985. "How to Have a Test Tube Baby." *Glamour*, May: 122-128.

Blank, R. 1985. "The Infertility Epidemic." *The Futurist* 19(1):17.

Bustillo, M. et al. 1984. "Nonsurgical Ovum Transfer As a Treatment in Infertile Women." *Journ. Amer. Med. Assoc.* 251, No. 9, pp. 1171-1173.

Center for Disease Control. 1982. "Infertility-United States." *Morbidity and Mortality Weekly Report* 34(14):197-199.

Davin, D. 1985. "The Single Child Family Policy in the Countryside," pp. 62-63 in *China's One-Child Family Policy*, edited by Elizabeth Croll, Delia Davin and Penny Kane. New York: St. Martin's Press.

Grobstein, C., M. Flower, and J. Mendeloff. 1983. "External Human Fertilization: An Evaluation of Policy." *Science* 222:127-133.

Hammer, R. E., R. D. Palmiter and R. L. Brinster. 1984. "Partial Correction of Murine Hereditary Growth Disorder by Germ-line Transportation of a New Gene." *Nature* 311:65-67.

Heape, W. 1891. "Preliminary Note On The Transplantation and Growth of Mammalian Ova Within A Uterine Foster-Mother." Proceedings of the Royal Society 48:457-458.

Horstadius, S. and A. Wolsky. 1936. "Studien Uber die Determination der Bilateral-symmetrie des jungen Seeigelkiemes." Roux Arch. 135:69-113.

McBain, J. C. and A. Trounson. 1984. "Patient Management-Treatment Cycle." pp. 49-65 in Clinical In Vitro Fertilization, edited by Carl Wood and Alan Trounson. New York: Springer-Verlag.

Miller, J. A. 1984. "Diagnostic DNA." Science News 126:104-107.

Milunsky, A. 1979. "The Prenatal Diagnosis of Chromosome Disorders," p. 96 in Genetic Disorders and the Fetus, edited by Aubrey Milunsky. New York: Plenum Press.

Mintz, B. 1962. "Formation of Geneotypically Mosaic Mouse Embryos." American Zoologist 2:432.

Mittenthal, S. 1984. "Amniocentesis on the Increase." New York Times, Aug. 25 (Section III): 1.

Mohr, L. and A. Trounson. 1984. In Vitro Fertilization and Embryo Growth." pp. 99-116 in Clinical In Vitro Fertilization, edited by Carl Wood and Alan Trounson. New York: Springer-Verlag.

Rosenwaks, Z., L. L. Veeck, and H. C. Liu. 1986. "Pregnancy Following Transfer of In Vitro Fertilized Donated Oocytes." Fertility and Sterility 45(3):417-20.

Rothberg, L. 1986. "Choosing The Sex of Your Baby," Woman's Newspaper, P. O. Box 1303, Princeton, N. J. 08542, May: Al.

Schneider, K. 1987. "New Animal Forms Will Be Patented" The New York Times April 17:1.

Short, R. V. 1977. "The Discovery of the Ovaries." pp. 1-39 in The Ovaries, 2nd edition, vol. 1, edited by S. Zuckermann and B. J. Weir. New York: Academic Press.

Steptoe, P. C. and R. G. Edwards. 1978. "Birth After The Re-Implantation of a Human Embryo." Lancet (Aug 12):366.

Tarkowski, A. J. 1964. "Patterns of Pigmentation in Experimentally Produced Mouse Chimaerae." J. Embryol. Exp. Morph. 12:575.

Trounson, A. 1986. "Preservation of Human Eggs and Embryos." Fertility and Sterility 46(1):1-12.

Trounson, A. and L. Mohr. 1983. "Human Pregnancy Following Cryopreservation, Thawing and Transfer of an Eight Cell Embryo," Nature 305:707.

Trounson, A. et al. 1981. "Pregnancies in Humans by Fertilization In Vitro and Embryo Transfer in the Controlled Ovulatory Cycle." Science 212:681-682.

Westoff, C. F. and R. R. Rindfuss. 1974. "Sex Pre-Selection in the United States: Some Implications," Science 184, pp. 633-636.

In Vitro Fertilization, GIFT and Related Technologies — Hope in a Test Tube

Patricia M. McShane

SUMMARY. *In vitro* fertilization (IVF) is demanding, expensive and inefficient. Nevertheless, tens of thousands of couples have undertaken the procedure because of their intense desire to have a biological child. Modifications of the current IVF process — simplification of ovulation induction and prediction of successful cycles; use of ultrasound instead of laparoscopy for egg retrieval; freezing of excess embryos for later replacement; and the substitution of GIFT (gamete intra-fallopian transfer) for IVF when it is indicated — may increase its acceptability to couples and improve success rates. Meanwhile, IVF has had tremendous impact on our understanding of fertility and should help physicians in their approach to infertility in the future. It has also ushered in a new era of genetic engineering whose potential we have not yet begun to realize.

HUMAN FERTILITY AND INFERTILITY

It is estimated that there are almost 3 million infertile couples in the United States, and the cost of infertility-related physician visits alone, not including surgery or medication, is estimated at over $200 million annually (Center for Disease Control 1985). Although the annual number of visits to physicians for infertility has more than doubled since 1980, there is in fact little data to support the popular notion that infertility is increasing. A recent population

---

Reprint request address: Patricia M. McShane, MD, Department of Obstetrics and Gynecology, Brigham and Women's Hospital, 75 Francis Street, Boston, Massachusetts 02115.

study showed that infertility rates adjusted for the woman's age are about the same as they were in 1965 (Center for Disease Control 1985). It is clear, however, that many couples are delaying child-bearing into their 30s, a time at which fertility is declining.

Peak fertility in women occurs between ages 20 to 29. The decreased birth rate after age 30 primarily reflects decreasing sexual activity and use of contraceptives. However, it is clear from a number of studies with fertility treatments such as ovulation induction and artificial insemination that reproductive success declines slowly with advancing age as well (Federation CECOS et al. 1982).

A fact not often appreciated by infertile couples is that the average probability of conception in a given menstrual cycle (fecundability) is estimated to be only 0.15 to 0.2 (Cramer et al. 1979). This is the basis for the definition of infertility as "one year of unprotected intercourse without conception." By one year, almost 85% of couples will have conceived, and those who have not conceived have a decreased chance in the second year. Although it is sometimes not possible to determine the cause of infertility or subfertility (long interval to conception), a careful investigation will uncover a problem in the woman, the man or both in over 90% of cases (Glass 1985).

The essential components of fertility are: ovulation; presence of competent sperm in sufficient numbers at the site of fertilization; and at least one Fallopian tube capable of picking up the egg, allowing fertilization and transporting the embryo into a uterus responsive to hormonal priming. The detection of ovulation has undergone considerable changes in recent years because of the availability of ultrasound to visualize the developing egg follicle and rapid urinary methods to detect the preovulatory surge of luteinizing hormone (LH) from the pituitary gland. Most of the time the tried and true method of basal body temperature charting to detect ovulation is sufficient though. If a woman is not ovulating because of abnormalities in the brain, pituitary gland or ovary itself, the use of ovulation induction agents results in a pregnancy in half the cases within a year. This is one of the most common and easily treated forms of infertility.

Deficiencies in sperm number, motility or quality of progression are seen in 30 to 40% of infertile couples (Glass 1985). These problems are more difficult to diagnose and treat. First of all, there is a continuum of pregnancy success rates such that a man with a sperm count of 5 million could not be said to be absolutely infertile, although his expectation of producing a pregnancy is about half that of a man with a count of 20 million. The same observation could be made about the other measures of sperm quality, which has made the definition of male infertility controversial, and the study of proposed therapies very difficult. Furthermore, very little is known about the basic processes of sperm transport through the female reproductive tract, sperm metabolism and the multiple functions involved in sperm recognition, penetration and junction with the egg. In some cases, there are hormonal or anatomic factors in the man which can be treated, resulting in increased fertility. More frequently, none of these factors are found. Treatment options for idiopathic male factor infertility are limited and the success rate is fairly low.

Anatomic derangements of the tubes and pelvis are becoming increasingly common and are among the most difficult to treat of women's fertility problems. Tubal infections (pelvic inflammatory disease or PID) are a common problem in young women and have resulted in an epidemic of tubal pregnancies and infertility. Another common condition resulting in varying degrees of pelvic pain, menstrual cramps and/or infertility is endometriosis. In this condition, tissue from the interior surface of the uterus (endometrium) gains access to the pelvis, most likely by flowing through the tubes at the time of menstruation. Often endometriosis will result in marked distortion of the anatomy because of scarring (adhesion formation), but even when adhesions are not present reduced fertility is observed. Hysterosalpingogram (X-ray of the uterus and tubes) and laparoscopy (surgical procedure to view the pelvis) are used for diagnosis. Less common causes of infertility include abnormal cervical mucus or sperm/cervical mucus interactions, uterine problems such as fibroids, and anomalies associated with prenatal exposure to DES (diethylstilbesterol).

There have been major advances in the use of medication (such as danazol) to treat endometriosis and some progress in the surgical approach to adhesions and tubal obstruction due to both infection and endometriosis. But these are still the most difficult category of fertility problems and were the original reasons for the development of *in vitro* fertilization. For example, one fertility unit reports that over a 2 year period, infertile couples with ovulation disorders achieved approximately 60% pregnancy rates; over 35% pregnancies for those with male infertility, but only 25% success for women with tubal damage or endometriosis (Collins et al. 1984). When no cause for infertility could be found, over 50% of the couples were able to achieve a pregnancy. Tubal factor infertility is the most common reason for using IVF, followed by male infertility, unexplained infertility, and cervical or immunological factors.

IN VITRO *FERTILIZATION PROCEDURES*

The accomplishment in 1978 of a normal birth following fertilization of the egg outside the body was the culmination of decades of reproductive research coupled with several new technologies: radioimmunoassay (RIA) to measure hormone levels rapidly; ultrasound imaging of the pelvis; and laparoscopy to remove eggs without major surgery. In the decade following this immense accomplishment, there have been a number of refinements to the basic approach taken by Drs. Robert Edwards and Patrick Steptoe in Bourn Hall, England. The success rate has steadily risen and hundreds of clinics have sprung up all over the world, resulting in several thousand births. Few centers have achieved even 10% pregnancy rates per cycle consistently, however, and the most successful large clinics report pregnancy rates below 20% when all patient groups are considered. Although simple in concept, success with IVF demands utmost dedication and attention to detail at every step in the process. These steps are: ovulation induction; egg harvest; addition of washed sperm to the eggs; and replacement of embryos into the uterus.

The major determinant of pregnancy rates with IVF is the number of embryos replaced into the uterus (Fishel et al. 1985; Jones et al. 1984; Wood et al. 1985). Three to four embryos seem to yield maximum pregnancy rates with acceptable numbers of multiple births. For this reason, the natural menstrual cycle with the production of a single egg has been abandoned and ovulation induction agents are used to stimulate development of multiple oocytes.

There are two drugs which are the mainstay of ovulation induction — clomiphene (Clomid, Serophene) and human menopausal gonadotropins (Pergonal). They can be used singly but are often used in combination. Each has a proven record of efficacy and safety when given to anovulatory women with careful monitoring. When used for normally ovulating women, ultrasound imaging of the pelvis reveals induction of at least two preovulatory follicles in three quarters of patients. About a quarter of patients will respond either with only one egg, fail to respond, or undergo premature spontaneous ovulation. Most women will achieve successful ovulation induction after several trials or after a change in medications.

Estrogen is the primary hormone of the follicular (oocyte maturation) phase of the menstrual cycle; rising levels reflect the activity of the ovary in the process of egg maturation. One enhancement in the art of ovulation induction for IVF is the recognition that certain levels and patterns of estrogen rise show strong correlation with pregnancy rates following IVF. Estrogen levels in blood are usually used in concert with ultrasound monitoring to determine the best timing for administration of hCG (human chorionic gonadotropin). This hormone is closely related chemically to LH (luteinizing hormone), the pituitary hormone which initiates ovulation. Approximately 34 to 36 hours after hCG administration, egg retrieval is carried out. This usually occurs around the 13th day of the menstrual cycle.

Laparoscopy is the predominant means of egg retrieval for IVF. With the women under general anesthesia, a needle is placed into her abdomen just below the umbilicus. Carbon dioxide gas is released into the abdomen, creating a space between the abdominal wall and the other abdominal contents. Then the laparoscope, a fiberoptic instrument about 1/2 inch (10 mm) in diameter, is introduced which enables the contents of the pelvis to be viewed easily. Several additional small incisions are made in the lower abdomen for grasping instruments and needles. When an ovary containing an egg follicle is visualized and stabilized, the follicle is punctured with a needle, suction is applied and the contents of the follicle collected in a tube or trap. This is then handed off the surgical field to a team of trained technicians and reproductive biologists, who rapidly scan the fluid under a microscope for the egg. A mature oocyte encircled with its nurturing granulosa cells can be identified quickly; immature oocytes are more difficult to see and may take several minutes, or longer if blood is present. An egg can be recovered from about 70% of the follicles. In some cases, the pelvic adhesions for which the woman requires IVF are so severe that none or only a small part of the ovary or ovaries can be seen and safely punctured. This may result in failure to obtain eggs in a small percent of cases. The mean number of eggs obtained using laparoscopy is between three and four, although over a dozen can sometimes be found.

A newer method of oocyte retrieval uses ultrasound guidance, which requires less anesthesia. The egg follicles can be easily "seen" through sound waves going through the bladder. With local anesthesia or light general anesthesia, a needle can be placed parallel to the ultrasound beam and tracked on its path into the follicle (Lenz and Lauritsen 1982; Wikland et al. 1983). Other approaches involve placing the needle into the bladder or vagina with abdominal ultrasound scanning (Gleicher et al. 1983; Parson et al. 1985). Most recently, ultrasound probes have been designed for placement in the vagina; the needle can then be passed along the path of the beam a short distance into the ovarian follicles (Dellenbach et al. 1985; Feichtinger and Kemeter 1986). The ultrasound procedure can be performed in an outpatient setting, it is well accepted by patients, and it generally costs less than laparoscopy. IVF centers with considerable experience using these techniques report pregnancy rates which are similar to those using the laparoscopy approach.

Approximately three quarters of the eggs obtained by these methods will appear mature under the microscope. Their appearance is identical to eggs retrieved in a natural cycle just prior to spontaneous ovulation. The remainder of the eggs will be either immature, degenerating or indeterminate. The heterogeneity of the oocyte population probably reflects the biology of egg selection in the natural and stimulated cycle. Because of intrinsic ovarian rhythms, it may be impossible to obtain a population of synchronous eggs regardless of our mastery of the endocrinology of the menstrual cycle (Chikazawa et al. 1986).

A few hours after egg harvest, the husband is asked to provide a sperm sample. The sperm are then carefully washed by gentle centrifugation in a physiological medium to remove the seminal plasma. By a variety of techniques, the most active fraction of sperm are separated and these are then counted and added to the eggs in separate culture dishes. Mature eggs are inseminated and placed in an incubator the afternoon of the egg retrieval; immature eggs are allowed to mature in a culture medium for up to 24 hours before insemination. The morning after the egg retrieval and insemination, the eggs are observed for signs of fertilization, i. e., the presence of male and female pronuclei in the middle of the cell and the extrusion of the extra genetic material in the form of a small polar body located alongside the cell membrane. These pronuclear eggs are then returned to the incubator for another 24 hours. On the second morning after egg retrieval, the embryos are now observed to have cleaved into 2, 4 or even 8 cells. At this time, they are replaced into the uterus through the cervix by means of a small plastic catheter. This is usually a simple procedure requiring no anesthesia; the woman experiences minimal cramping and very little pain. Bedrest is then advised, usually for the remainder of the day or overnight in the hospital. Although technically simple in most cases, this is the point at which most IVF cycles do not succeed; most women will receive embryos, but few will become pregnant.

Following the embryo transfer, progesterone is usually administered until a pregnancy is established or until two weeks have elapsed and no pregnancy is detected by blood testing. Progesterone is the predominant hormone of the second half (luteal phase) of the menstrual cycle, and is known to affect the development of the uterine lining. Normal preparation of the endometrium is essential for embryo implantation and early pregnancy maintenance. Because of the high estrogen levels resulting from the hormonal ovulation induction, endometrial inadequacy can be seen in a number of women (Dlugi et al. 1985). Giving extra progesterone is thought to overcome this deficiency and improve pregnancy rates, but this has not been conclusively demonstrated.

The handling of the eggs and sperm in the culture laboratory requires extraordinary skill and attention to detail. Although we have learned a great deal in recent years about the biology of human gametes and embryos, the small amount of available material and ethical considerations have meant that most of what we know is extrapolated from mouse and other laboratory animal experiments. Currently, a mature human egg can be expected to undergo fertilization about 70% of the time. Once fertilization is achieved, 80% of these eggs will go to divide and are presumed to be normal. What little work has been done with "excess" human embryos has shown that a substantial minority of these embryos are actually not normal by biochemical, genetic or morphological criteria (Verlinsky and Pergament 1986); this may be the basis of low pregnancy success rates even with replacement of multiple "normal" embryos.

PREGNANCY OUTCOMES

It is essential to understand what criteria are used to establish the diagnosis of pregnancy in order to understand reported success rates and pregnancy outcomes in IVF programs (Jones et al. 1983). A small number of women will have biochemical evidence of pregnancy by blood testing, but will not experience more than a week or two delay in their menstrual bleeding. This is presumed to be a very early pregnancy which was not continued, either because of abnormalities of the placenta and embryo itself, or because of poor receptivity of the uterus. This is termed a "subclinical," "preclinical" or "biochemical" pregnancy. Most IVF centers do not include these pregnancies in their statistics.

If a woman is at least two weeks late for her menses with a positive pregnancy test (6 weeks pregnant), this is termed a pregnancy for the purpose of IVF statistics. Demonstration of tissue, either after removal of a tubal pregnancy or miscarriage, also meets criteria for establishment of a pregnancy. Only about two thirds of pregnancies in an IVF center will yield a surviving infant because of pregnancy loss in the first trimester (20-30% spontaneous abortion and 5% tubal pregnancy) (Andrews et al. 1985; Fishel et al. 1985); less commonly, premature labor or other obstetrical complications occur, especially in multiple pregnancy, leading to the delivery of a previable fetus or to a neonatal death. The incidence of such obstetrical complications may be slightly higher in IVF pregnancies than in the general obstetrical population. From a genetic and developmental perspective, IVF babies are no different than other babies; i.e., there is a risk of chromosome problems proportional to maternal age and a risk of major congenital malformation of about 2% (Andrews et al. 1985).

The overall rate of multiple birth is about 20% and is dependent on the number of embryos replaced in the uterus. Above three to four embryos, the rate of twins and triplets approaches 50% without appreciably raising the pregnancy rate (Jones et al. 1984).

SUCCESS RATES

IVF programs generally report two different statistics: pregnancies per egg retrieval procedure and pregnancies per patient having embryo transfer. The difference between the number of egg retrievals and the number of embryo transfers represents the number of cycles in which no eggs are obtained, or in which none of the eggs fertilize normally. By these measures, the average pregnancy rate in U.S. centers is thought to be about 7%. The larger centers usually report success rates in the teens when no patients or cycles are excluded (Fishel et al. 1985; Laufer et al. 1986; Wood et al. 1985). A few programs, usually with highly selected patients, report greater than 20% pregnancies. Unfortunately, it is not uncommon for IVF programs to mention their success rate "per patient" or other such statistic to the local newspaper, failing to mention that patients may have undergone more than one cycle (Soules 1985). Another misleading figure may be the success rate within a short time frame, since a month of many good outcomes may follow a long stretch with few pregnancies.

Patient selection and the cancellation rate per ovulation induction cycle undoubtedly contributes to the disparity in success rates between clinics, since age, diagnosis and hormonal response pattern are very important determinants of IVF success. But much of the disparity probably relates to the experience of the program, as well as the skill of the staff and many intangibles. The oldest and largest U.S. IVF center performed over 40 egg harvests before achieving a pregnancy; while much of the learning which was occurring in those pioneer efforts is now readily available in the medical literature, there is no substitute for first hand experience.

The Norfolk program has reported that their IVF success rate is essentially unchanged by the age of the woman up to the age of 40 (Jones et al. 1984), but Edwards' and Steptoe's Bourn Hall clinic and Wood and colleagues in the Monash program (Melbourne, Australia) reported the expected drop in pregnancy rates by 5 year age increments in 1679 patient cycles (Table I) and 1533 cycles respectively (Fishel et al. 1985; Wood et al. 1985). Most programs report that the patients most likely to achieve pregnancy through IVF are women whose infertility problem is either tubal factor or mild endometriosis (Table II) (Fishel et al. 1985; Wood et al. 1985). The major pitfall for these patients is limited ovarian accessibility. (A screening laparoscopy is sometimes performed to exclude from IVF programs women in whom there is little or no access to the ovaries); severe endometriosis is also often associated with inaccessible ovaries as well as decreased egg development. Unexplained infertility is regarded by some programs as a favorable diagnosis, but Steptoe recently reported a low success rate in this group. This may depend on differences in the definition of unexplained infertility and in the age of the patients.

When IVF is used to overcome male infertility (low sperm count and/or motility), lower rates of fertilization per oocyte usually result as well as failed fertilization in all the available eggs; in these cases, one generally expects pregnancy rates per laparoscopy to be half the rate for tubal factor infertility (Fishel et al. 1985; Wood et al. 1985). If fertilization is achieved, the pregnancy rate per embryo transfer is the same. Pregnancy rates when there is combined male

Table I

IVF Pregnancy and Abortion Rates by Age of Woman

(Adapted from Fishel SB, Edwards RG, et al: J In Vitro Fertil Embr Trans 2:123-131, 1985)

	Age		
	Less than 35	35-39	Over 39
Pregnancy rate	17%	13%	6%
Abortion rate	27%	34%	56%

Table II

IVF Success Rates by Infertility Diagnosis

(Adapted from Jones et al: Three years of IVF at Norfolk.
Fertil Steril 42(6):829, 1984)

Diagnosis	Patients	Cycles	Pregnancy Rate by Cycle	Pregnancy Rate by Transfer
			%	%
Tube	249	454	19	24
Male	23	30	10	27
Diethylstilbesterol	17	25	16	19
Endometriosis	11	20	30	40
Normal	11	18	28	38
Other	8	13	14	15
Total	319	560	19	25

and female infertility, or with the less common conditions such as immunological infertility, are usually lower than when tubal factor infertility alone is the problem.

Other determinants of success pertain to the woman's response to ovulation induction. There is now good evidence that a moderate rise of blood estrogen levels and a moderate amount of total estrogen are more favorable than either a high or low response pattern (Dirnfeld et al. 1985). Rising estradiol levels after the ovulatory dose of hCG also predict higher success rates (Laufer et al. 1986). Several groups have reported that the hCG should be given on the sixth day of the estradiol rise (Levran et al. 1985; Quigley et al. 1985). The hormonal patterns are generally not reflected in the recovery rate or the appearance of the eggs or embryos, again suggesting that there are subtle differences in egg and embryo quality, or effects on the endometrium, which we are thus far not able to detect. Information regarding optimum hormonal patterns has been helpful in refining ovulation induction and cancelling unfavorable cycles, but our ability to dramatically alter a woman's response is limited.

The most important cycle variable is the number of embryos transferred, which is a function of the ovarian response, number of eggs retrieved, fertilization and cleavage rates. A plateau in the pregnancy rate is observed when three to four embryos are replaced, while multiple pregnancy rates rise sharply (Fishel et al. 1985). This results in a dilemma for the IVF team: what to do with the excess eggs or embryos. The options are to discard them, donate them, perform research or freeze them.

FREEZING OF EGGS AND EMBRYOS

Currently the option most responsive to the needs of the couple is freezing of the excess embryos for replacement in a subsequent cycle (Trounson et al. 1986). The legal and ethical concerns arising from this are tremendous, and some states and countries have prohibited this practice. Unfortunately, mature eggs subjected to freezing and storage undergo extensive damage and have thus far not been able to produce pregnancies. Progress is being made in this area, however, and hopefully the process will be improved soon.

In centers where embryo freezing and embryo donation to other women have been used extensively, some interesting observations have been made which may modify our approach to IVF. Various programs have observed that an embryo is more likely to implant when transferred in a natural cycle, rather than one in which there has been intensive hormonal stimulation. For example, women who do not become pregnant after transfer of several embryos in their egg retrieval cycle have a higher success rate per embryo transfer when the frozen embryos are later replaced in a monitored but unstimulated cycle (Frydman et al. 1986). Similarly, donated embryos are more likely to produce pregnancies in the natural cycle of the recipient than similar embryos do in the stimulated cycle of the donor (Lutjen et al. 1986). This has prompted speculation that the major cause of failure in IVF cycles relates to the consequences of high hormone levels, and perhaps all embryos should be frozen for later transfer. This might greatly increase the efficiency of IVF.

Success in freezing eggs rather than embryos is likely to greatly reduce ethical concerns.

GIFT AND OTHER REPRODUCTIVE TECHNOLOGIES

Success with IVF has led to the development of the GIFT procedure (gamete intra-fallopian transfer) (Asch et al. 1986). The ovary is stimulated and eggs harvested by laparoscopy. Instead of allowing fertilization to occur in an incubator, prepared sperm are injected in tandem with three to four eggs a short distance into the end of the Fallopian tube, the site where fertilization occurs normally. The rationale for this procedure is the conjecture that several types of infertility may be due to failure of the egg and sufficient sperm to be present in the tube. Unexplained infertility may be due to failure of the tube to pick up the egg from the ovary. Male infertility or cervical infertility in women may mean that not enough sperm are present at the site of fertilization. Aside from the necessity of having at least one normal tube and the requirement for laparoscopy instead of ultrasound, the major disadvantage of GIFT is the inability to determine whether fertilization has occurred. The success rate of 25% is probably greater than the success rate of IVF, but the patient population is not comparable. Unpublished data thus far suggest that the pregnancy rate for cervical, unexplained, and immunological infertility is high, whereas the success rate for male infertility is low, confirming our impression from IVF that fertilization failure rather than gamete transport is the major defect.

Various forms of surrogacy have also evolved utilizing technologies related to IVF. Donor insemination for male infertility is well accepted and technically simple. Donor oocytes and embryos from IVF cycles, and oocytes obtained from volunteer women at the time of tubal sterilization operations, can now be given to women with inaccessible ovaries, absent ovaries, premature ovarian failure or genetic disease (Navot et al. 1986). Similarly, a normal fertile volunteer can undergo artificial insemination with the intended father's semen; flushing the uterus will yield a viable embryo in most cycles; this can then be placed into the uterus of the intended mother (Bustillo et al. 1984). Women with medical contraindications to pregnancy or who have had a hysterectomy or have no abnormal uterus can undergo IVF. Resulting embryos can be placed into the uterus of a willing surrogate for the remainder of the pregnancy. The expense of procedures involving surrogates is even higher than the cost of an IVF cycle, currently estimated at an average of $4,100 nationwide. The introduction of surrogacy, particularly if there are monetary incentives, raises a host of additional ethical concerns, and it is unlikely that these procedures will be widely accepted.

THE FUTURE OF REPRODUCTIVE TECHNOLOGY

The availability of human embryos in the lab has ushered in a "brave new world" of human genetics and reproduction. One procedure with obvious immediate clinical application is the injection of sperm into the egg to overcome fertilization failure (Lassalle et al. 1986). This often results in damage to the egg and no pregnancies have yet resulted. It is likely that this technique can be perfected in the near future, though.

Our ability to utilize embryos for genetic treatment is probably a number of years in the future, but sophisticated techniques with minute quantities of material can already be used for diagnosis of fatal or disabling genetic diseases, such as enzyme defects. One potential scenario would be removing one cell from a 4 or 8 cell embryo of a couple who have previously had a child affected with Tay-Sachs disease, for example, and freezing the embryo until a diagnosis could be confirmed. It seems unlikely that such involved, expensive and risky procedures would be used for frivolous applications, such as sex selection where no genetic disease is involved, but simplification of all the procedures would make this more likely.

Another potential application would be culturing normal tissue such as bone marrow or liver from more advanced embryos. This could be maintained in an organ bank for transplantation into children and adults needing the tissues. This possibility is hypothetical currently because we lack knowledge of the proper culture conditions for maintaining more advanced embryos and human tissues.

REFERENCES

Andrews, M. C. et al. 1985. "An Analysis of the Obstetric Outcome of 25 Consecutive Pregnancies Conceived *In Vitro* and Resulting in 100 Deliveries." *American Journal of Obstetrics and Gynecology* 154:848-54.

Asch, R. H. et al. 1986. "Preliminary Experiences with Gamete Intrafallopian Transfer (GIFT). *Fertility and Sterility* 45:366-70.

Bustillo, M. et al. 1984. "Nonsurgical Ovum Transfer as a Treatment in Infertile Women." *Journal of the American Medical Association* 251:1171-75.

Center for Disease Control 1985. "Infertility—United States, 1982." *Morbidity and Mortality Weekly Report* 14:197-207.

Chikazawa, K. et al. 1986. "Morphological and Endocrinological Studies on Follicular Development During the Human Menstrual Cycle." *Journal of Clinical Endocrinology and Metabolism* 62:305-10.

Collins, J. A. et al. 1984. "A Proportional Hazards Analysis of the Clinical Characteristics of Infertile Couples." *American Journal of Obstetrics and Gynecology* 148:527-32.

Cramer, D. W. et al. 1979. "Statistical Methods in Evaluating the Outcome of Infertility Therapy." *Fertility and Sterility* 21:80-6.

Dellenbach, P. et al. 1985. "Transvaginal Sonographically Controlled Follicle Puncture for Oocyte Retrieval." *Fertility and Sterility* 44:656-62.

Dirnfeld, M. et al. 1985. "Growth Rate of Follicular Estrogen Secretion in Relation to the Outcome of *In Vitro* Fertilization and Embryo Replacement." *Fertility and Sterility* 43:379-84.

Dlugi, A. M. et al. 1985. "Altered Follicular Development in Clomiphene Citrate Versus Human Menopausal Gonadotropin-Stimulated Cycles for *In Vitro* Fertilization." *Fertility and Sterility* 43:40-7.

Federation CECOS et al. 1982. "Female Fecundity as a Function of Age: Results of Artificial Insemination in 2193 Nulliparous Women with Azoospermic Husbands." *New England Journal of Medicine* 306:404-8.

Feichtinger, W. and Kemeter, P. 1986. "Transvaginal Sector Scan Sonography for Needle Guided Transvaginal Follicle Aspiration and Other Applications in Gynecologic Routine and Research." *Fertility and Sterility* 45:722-5.

Fishel, S. B. et al. 1985. "Implantation, Abortion and Birth after *In Vitro* Fertilization Using the Natural Menstrual Cycle or Follicular Stimulation with Clomiphene Citrate and Human Menopausal Gonadotrophin." *Journal of In Vitro Fertilization and Embryo Transfer* 2:123-31.

Frydman, R. et al. 1986. "Programmed Oocyte Retrieval During Routine Laparoscopy and Embryo Cryopreservation for Later Transfer." *American Journal of Obstetrics and Gynecology* 155:122-7.

Glass, R. H. 1985. "Infertility." Pp. in *Reproductive Endocrinology: Physiology, Pathophysiology and Clinical Management*, edited by S.S.C. Yen and R.B. Jaffe. Philadelphia: W.B. Saunders, p. 575.

Gleicher, N. et al. 1983. "Egg Retrieval for *In Vitro* Fertilization by Sonographically Controlled Vaginal Culdocentesis." *Lancet* 2:508.

Jones, H. W. et al. 1983. "What is a Pregnancy? A Question for Programs of *In Vitro* Fertilization." *Fertility and Sterility* 40:728-31.

Jones, H. W. et al. 1984. "Three Years of *In Vitro* Fertilization at Norfolk." *Fertility and Sterility* 42:826-34.

Lassalle, B. et al. 1986. "*In Vitro* Fertilization of Hamster and Human Oocytes by Microinjection of Sperm." *Journal of In Vitro Fertilization and Embryo Transfer* 3:69-73.

Laufer, N. et al. 1986. "The Association Between Preovulatory Serum 17-Estradiol Pattern and Conception in Human Menopausal Gonadotropin-Human Chorionic Gonadotropin Stimulation." *Fertility and Sterility* 46:73-80.

Lenz, S. and Lauritsen, J. G. 1982. "Ultrasonically Guided Percutaneous Aspiration of Human Follicles Under Local Anaesthesia: A New Method of Collecting Oocytes for *In Vitro* Fertilization." *Fertility and Sterility* 39:673-7.

Levran, D. et al. 1985. "Analysis of the Outcome of *In Vitro* Fertilization in Relation to the Timing of Human Chorionic Gonadotropin Administration on the Duration of Estradiol Rise in Stimulated Cycles." *Fertility and Sterility* 44:335-40.

Lutjen, P. J. et al. 1986. "The Australian Method of Embryo and Oocyte Donation." *Journal of In Vitro Fertilization and Embryo Transfer* 3:69-71.

Navot, D. et al. 1986. "Artificially Induced Endometrial Cycles and Establishment of Pregnancies in the Absence of Ovaries." *New England Journal of Medicine* 314:806-11.

Parson, J. et al. 1985. "Oocyte Retrieval of *In Vitro* Fertilization by Ultrasonically Guided Needle Aspiration Via the Urethra." *Lancet* 1:1076-7.

Quigley, M. M. et al. 1985. "Timing Human Chorionic Gonadotropin Administration by Days of Estradiol Rise." *Fertility and Sterility* 44:791-5.

Soules, M. R. 1985. "The IVF Pregnancy Rate: Lets Be Honest with One Another." *Fertility and Sterility* 43:511-2.

Trounson, A. 1986. "Preservation of Human Eggs and Embryos." *Fertility and Sterility* 46:1-8.

Verlinsky, Y. and Pergament, E. 1986. "Genetic Analysis of Human Embryos Prior to Implantation." *Journal of In Vitro Fertilization and Embryo Transfer* 3:83.

Wikland, M. et al. 1983. "Collection of Human Oocytes by the Use of Sonography." *Fertility and Sterility* 39:603-8.

Wood, C. et al. 1985. "Factors Influencing Pregnancy Rates Following *In Vitro* Fertilization and Embryo Transfer." *Fertility and Sterility* 43:245-50.

Fetal Imaging
and Fetal Monitoring:
Finding the Ethical Issues

Caroline Whitbeck

SUMMARY. Ethical issues are raised in connection with three technologies used to detect abnormalities or distress in the fetus in late pregnancy and during labor: (1) Ultrasound for fetal diagnosis, a technology used with increasing frequency in pregnancy and labor and one which some are advocating for *routine* use in pregnancy; (2) The newest of the imaging technologies, magnetic resonance imaging (MRI), which is not now commonly used for fetal imaging, but may soon be; (3) The electronic fetal monitors, some of which work by application of the physical principles of ultrasound behavior and raise many of the same ethical issues.

This paper argues that women-centered critiques of birthing technologies augment the concern with the health risks posed by those technologies with concerns about the risks that they pose to human relationships.

Although IVF and other dramatic technological interventions in procreation and birth are getting much media attention, the less dramatic but commonly used technologies of ultrasound imaging and fetal monitoring have at least as great a potential for changing the birth process and women's lives. In this respect they are like amniocentesis and other commonly used techniques for prenatal diagnosis in the first two trimesters, which Rayna Rapp discusses elsewhere.

Ethical issues arise concerning the technologies used to detect

The research for this paper was supported by grant 94159 from the National Science Foundation.

47

fetal abnormality or distress in late pregnancy and during labor. The two imaging technologies I shall discuss are:

1. Ultrasound for fetal diagnosis, a technology used with increasing frequency in pregnancy and labor and one which some are advocating for routine use in pregnancy.
2. The newest of the imaging technologies, magnetic resonance imaging, MRI—formerly called "nuclear magnetic imaging," before the word "nuclear" began to make people uncomfortable—is only now beginning to be used for fetal imaging in a few special cases, but may come to be used much more commonly. It raises many of the same issues as ultrasound, but differs in that it is a technology with *very* high fixed costs, and this factor is very likely to affect the pressures for and against its use in pregnancy. I shall also briefly discuss a third technology which, like ultrasound imaging, is commonly used and which raises many of the same ethical issues:
3. The fetal monitor. Fetal monitors are devices for monitoring the fetal heart rate and uterine contractions rate and making a continuous recording on a polygraph.

My intention is not merely to enumerate ethical issues raised by the three technologies, but to draw attention to some differences in the way in which these ethical issues are identified. There are different perspectives on what is *valuable* or even what is *usual* in human life. When we use these different frameworks of assumptions and commitments, certain risks stand out and others may be obscured. Therefore, the question of just what the ethical issues are is significant. Women-centered critiques of reproductive technology provide a model for an expanded critique of other medical technologies and, indeed, for a more adequate assessment of the impact of *all* technology.

Ultrasound imaging of the fetus uses sound waves of frequencies higher than the audible range that are sent into the abdomen of the pregnant woman. The sound waves are reflected at rates which depend on the density of the body part. The reflected waves are converted into electronic signals from which an image is then constructed. Several types of devices have been used for ultrasound imaging. The earliest of these created a static picture. The type of ultrasound that is most commonly used today is a so-called "real-time" device that uses rapid, pulsed sound waves to create a moving image of the fetus.

Ultrasound is commonly used in "external fetal monitors" and in certain hand-held devices for making fetal heart tones audible. In all types of fetal monitors, what is produced is not an image, but audio signals that make fetal heart sounds audible. There are two basic types of fetal monitor: the external or indirect monitor mentioned above, and the internal or direct fetal monitor. The indirect or external device is the more frequently used. It is "clinically non-invasive" — which is to say that it does not require any cutting or insertion of material into the tissue of the woman or fetus — and may be used before labor begins. The ultrasound transducer, which is made of a transmitting and receiving crystal, is placed on the woman's abdomen and held in place with a belt. Jelly or mineral oil is used to facilitate the transmission of sound waves between the transducer and the abdomen. This technique requires the woman to lie on her back and be relatively immobile.

The direct or internal fetal monitor has electrodes that are "attached to" the baby's scalp. (Actually they penetrate the baby's scalp to a depth of 2 mm.) The procedure therefore requires that the membranes containing the baby and the amniotic fluid be ruptured in order to expose the baby's scalp; to avoid the risk of infection to the baby, labor must be induced if it has not already begun. Ultrasound imaging and the fetal monitor are both diagnostic technologies that are used primarily in late pregnancy or during the birth process.

Reservations about the routine use of fetal ultrasound most commonly revolve around questions of safety. For example, at the end of a recent article, "Biological Effects of Ultrasound" (Statmeyer and Christman 1982, 78), the authors conclude that more information is needed about the effects of ultrasound, that the potential for acute adverse effects has not been systematically studied and that the potential for delayed effects has virtually been ignored. Because of the difficulties in conducting the requisite studies, they recommend an interim policy of using ultrasound only if warranted by clear diagnostic benefit to the patient.

The absence of systematic studies of adverse effects, especially of delayed adverse effects, is of course even more true when MRI is used for fetal imaging. In MRI the image is obtained from information gained by subjecting the patient to a gradient magnetic field about 10,000 times the strength of the earth's field and measuring the relaxation time of the hydrogen carbon or nitrogen nuclei as they remit absorbed energy. The gulf between the assertion that there are "no known hazards" and the assertion that a technology is *known to be safe* in specified applications is enormous, especially for a hitherto unused technology like MRI.

The American College of Obstetrics and Gynecology itself recommends against routine use of ultrasound in pregnancies, largely because its risks are uncertain. The lack of data about the biological effects of ultrasound, and the uncertain value of its routine use in pregnancy are sufficient to justify limiting the application of this technology.

However, the issue of the physical safety of women and fetuses, and the requirement to inform patients of uncertainty about the hazards, is not the only ethically significant consequence of the use of this technology. We need also to consider the effect of information about the fetus, together with the effects of its mode of presentation upon the human relationships involved. Beyond the question of the biological risks posed by these technologies (risks that may not be outweighed by the risks posed by the conditions that they detect) is the question of how these technologies direct our attention to certain types of physical risks and away from other matters. In particular, we need to find out the extent to which technologies lead us to ignore human stories and the human relationships that are deeply affected by the birth experience. The concern has been well-expressed by Dianne Patychuck, writing on the use of fetal imaging with ultrasound. She asks whether these technologies can be used "without driving a wedge between women and their future children" (Patychuck 1985). The most common argument against use of the fetal monitor is that it is frequently misused or misinterpreted, so that normal deliveries are taken to be problematic. As a consequence, unnecessary caesarean deliveries are performed which result in increased morbidity and even mortality. These concerns are included by Haverkamp and Orleans (1982) in their enumeration of the negative effects of the use of the fetal monitor:

1. EFM increases cesarean sections, some unnecessary, for reasons of fetal distress and dystocia.
2. EFM patterns are not easy to read:
   a. Normal or reassuring FHR [fetal heart rate] patterns are sometimes miscalled ominous.
   b. Subtle ominous patterns can be missed.
3. Ominous FHR patterns overcall fetal distress, for example, as with late decelerations where only 30% of infants may be acidotic, whereas 70% are normal.
4. Monitors restrict patient movement. EFM, especially external monitors, tend to force patients to remain flat on their backs in labor.
5. Monitors seem to, but should not, replace nurses as caregivers in labor.
6. The monitor becomes the focus for partners, nurses, and physicians rather than the woman in labor.
7. The monitor medicalizes labor and appears to interfere with freedom, relaxation, and motion, producing what some have called negative biofeedback of anxiety that tends to interrupt labor. (Haverkamp and Orleans 1982, 131)

The three women-centered critiques deserve special attention. The risk that the fetal monitor will inappropriately replace the nurse is the first concern. More explicitly, this is the concern that essential human relationships will be lost. Two other concerns, about the restriction of motion required by the external monitors, and about the medicalization of labor and production of anxiety, hint at a similar risk. The risk is trivialized if it is interpreted as a small increase in discomfort to the pregnant woman. The issue is that of treating the birthing woman as what is commonly called "clinical material," robbing her of her agency and her opportunity to act on behalf of her baby. This endangers the maternal-child relationship, which appears to be integral to the identity of both the mother and child. The problem of the medicalization of childbirth would be comparable to intimidating or drugging a bride and groom and having competent professionals say their wedding vows for them. It would still be possible to have a good marriage after such an experience, but the experience itself would be an injury from which the couple would have to recover.

Consideration of the influence of technologies on human relationships takes as its starting point the recognition of the social nature of human life and the dynamic character of the moral self. A notable illustration of a women-centered examination of diagnostic reproductive technologies that takes this approach is Barbara Katz Rothman's study of the effects of amniocentesis on the relationship between a woman and her fetus and later her child. In her book *The Tentative Pregnancy: Prenatal Diagnosis and the Future of Motherhood*, she focuses on the relationship of a woman to her fetus as the initial phase of the relationship of a mother to her child:

> A diagnostic technology that pronounces judgement halfway through pregnancy makes extraordinary demands on women to separate themselves from the fetus within. Rather than moving from complete attachment through the separation that only just begins at birth, this technology demands that we begin with separation and distancing. Only after an acceptable judgment has been declared, only after the fetus is deemed worthy of keeping, is attachment to begin. (Rothman 1986: 114)

As I have argued elsewhere, concern with the quality of relationships, and with the development of people in and through their relationships, reflects a perspective that is distinct from both modern individualism and traditional patriarchy (Whitbeck 1984). In drawing our attention to the effect on human relationships, women-centered critiques of reproductive technology provide a model for an expanded critique of other medical technology and, indeed, for a more adequate assessment of the impact of all technology. Concerns about the medicalization of childbirth, the "disempowerment" of birthing women, and the "commodification of life" figures prominently in the work of many feminists—for example: Gena Corea *The Mother Machine*, essays in the collections *Birth*

Control and Controlling Birth and *The Custom-Made Child?*
(Holmes, Hoskins & Gross 1981a & 1981b), and *Test Tube Women*
(Arditti, Klein & Minden 1984). These concerns have distinguished
women-centered critiques of birthing technology. In the evaluation
of ultrasound imaging and the fetal monitor, women-centered critiques raise the question of how these technologies influence human
relationships and the capacity to fulfill responsibility, and augment
concerns about biological safety and informed consent.

It is important to question the common assumption that biological
safety necessarily takes precedence over questions of human relationships, and moral integrity. It is only if we accept the belief that
(correctly designed and employed) technology can solve the peren-
nial problems of death and physical suffering — that it can *in principle* provide immortality and invulnerability — that giving precedence to assuring biological well-being over relationships and
moral integrity seems at all plausible. Since everyone dies sooner or
later, and our physical well-being is always at risk, questions of
moral integrity and whether our lives make sense are not easily
relegated to second place.

Women-centered critiques share some concerns with critiques offered by certain religious groups, but there are major differences in
the central focus of the criticisms. Like women-centered critiques,
religious criticisms warn against the overreliance on technology and
the intrusion of market values in assessments of medical technology. Although some religious groups emphasize the issue of con-
science (moral integrity), their best known criticisms focus on the
prohibition of such acts as the use of contraception, donor insemination, and abortion. They are objected to on the grounds either that
human intervention in those areas of life is religiously proscribed
and will corrupt the individual and society, or that there is an absolute prohibition on the particular acts or their foreseeable consequences (e.g., feticide). This focus on particular acts contrasts with
the women-centered focus on the quality of human relationships
and people's capacity to fulfill the responsibilities of their relationships and thereby maintain moral integrity.

One of the few other sources of evaluation of medical technologies in terms of their influence on human relationships has come
from those concerned with death and dying, although assessments

in medical ethics of "high technology dying" have tended to focus on dignity rather than on relationships, responsibility, and moral integrity. An interesting example of recent work that *has* focused on the consequences of life-support technology for relationships and responsibility, from a psychological point of view, is a study of bereavement by Parkes and Weiss. The authors discuss one of their subjects, a bereaved wife who performed much of her husband's care, in the following way: "In a paradoxical fashion, the very absence of an efficient medical machine which would have taken over his care and deprived her of this opportunity, may have aided her eventual recovery. There is a real danger that intensive care units and other inpatient facilities, to the extent that they take away from the family the opportunity to care for the dying individual, may create problems for the family in the future" (Parkes & Weiss 1983:96).

It is important to emphasize that the concerns about relationship and moral integrity themselves augment, and are not independent of, considerations about physical safety, since one aspect of a person's moral responsibility toward another is to safeguard the other's physical well-being. Women-centered critiques share concerns about biological safety with other technological assessments.

Several trends concerning birthing technology bear watching in light of the concerns both about relationships, responsibility and moral integrity, and about physical safety. The first of these are concerns about inequities of access to medical technology, distribution of health care resources and the displacement of an understanding of human relationships by market models — the "commodification of life" that occurs in other areas as well as medicine. Such commodification is very much in evidence in legal circles where advocates of so-called "law and economics" thinking advocate eliminating "economically inefficient" adoption agencies and legalizing the sale of babies (Barrett, 1986).

The refusal of health insurers and other third party payers to underwrite the *routine* use of ultrasound has been a factor countering the trend to subject patients to the unknown long-term risks of this procedure unnecessarily. At the same time, the feminization of poverty, together with the replacement of the 1960's concern with fair distribution of health care resources by the 1980's concern with cost containment, has meant that many women do not have access to needed medical technology.

Because of the large number of births each year, there are particular financial incentives for some parties to promote the use of new technologies with high fixed costs as appropriate for use in pregnancy and childbirth without sufficient regard for the special biological vulnerability of infants, the emotional vulnerability of birthing women, or the importance of the mother-infant bond. For example, a recent presentation at M.I.T. on magnetic resonance imaging (MRI) made much of the fact that because MRI employs non-ionizing radiation, it does not pose many of the risks associated with other imaging technologies used to detect neurological or cardiac injury. For this reason, it is said to be "non-invasive" even though there is little or no knowledge about its long-term biological effects. One faculty member pointed out that to justify the huge fixed cost of the device, MRI would have to be used with more than neurological and cardiac patients. He urged the presenter to look to pregnant women as a "huge potential market" for MRI.

In addition to the use of market models, we find an equally dangerous tendency to "do everything possible," which includes some possibilities that turn out, from the patient's point of view, to be better left unexplored. My observation from working and teaching at six hospitals and medical schools is that this error is common both among health care providers and patient's families. A provider may tell a patient or family that some procedure is "your only hope" meaning that it represents the only hope, however slim, of postponing death for a significant period. Of course, there are other things the patient might hope for, such as to die at home surrounded by one's family relatively free of pain and anxiety rather than in a hospital surrounded by bright lights and machines. The provider's tendency to think first of the actions that he or she was trained to take may become so entrenched that patients are thought of as mere "clinical material," i.e., as merely the occasion for clinical action.

Debate over what constitutes an inappropriately high level of care has received the most media attention in cases in which life support technology is applied with little hope of the patient's recovery. "Baby Doe" cases of severely impaired newborns fall within this high visibility group. The danger of an inappropriately high level of care—at least for those who can pay for it—exists in many other areas, too, such as infertility, prenatal, and birthing care. In these cases we need to ask: When are we better off not knowing? Are we obliged to acquire all prognostic information? What kinds of support do people need in order to face new decisions? When is it reasonable and/or responsible to simply accept some impairment (such as infertility) and get on with the rest of one's life?

The tendencies to think of patients as potential markets, or to unthinkingly treat them as clinical material, represents a special threat to women in a society that demonstrates some particularly callous and destructive attitudes towards women and women's bodies. Against the grim background of the huge pornography industry and other evidence of social misogyny, it becomes important to resist the tendency to use technology in ways that turns attention away from the woman in labor, or which devalues the pregnant woman's own felt experience of the fetus, in favor of publicly observable images on a cathode ray tube. A dramatic illustration of the tendency to devalue the woman's experience in favor of a publicly observable image is given by Becky Sarah in the example of the Boston obstetrician who subjects her patients to ultrasound imaging every month of pregnancy for the purpose of "helping the woman bond to her baby."

The relationship of a woman to her fetus and to her baby seems increasingly unintelligible to our culture. Technologies that provide prenatal and birthing information threaten to transform the relationship between a woman and her fetus into a market or adversarial one. The potential for such transformation is aptly illustrated by the headline of a recent article in the *Wall Street Journal* on prenatal care: "WOMEN'S RIGHTS vs. FETAL RIGHTS LOOMS AS THORNY AND DIVISIVE ISSUE" (Otten 1985).

In summary, women-centered critiques of reproductive technology consider not only risks posed to biological well-being, but also risks posed to human relationships and to moral integrity. It is not surprising that women-centered critiques have led the way in this area since in our individualistic society the care and tending of relationships—"the making and mending of social life" as Peggy McIntosh calls it—has been left to women. Risk to relationships and to integrity constitutes a dimension that must be incorporated into our assessment of technology.

REFERENCES

Arditti, R.; Klein, R. D.; Minden, S. 1984. *Test-Tube Women*. Boston: Pandora Press.

Barrett, P. M. "A Movement Called 'Law and Economics' Sways Legal Circles," *Wall Street Journal*, August 4, 1986, 1.

Corea, G. 1985. *The Mother Machine: Reproductive Technologies from Artificial Insemination to Artificial Wombs*. New York: Harper and Row.

Haverkamp, A. & Orleans M. 1982. "An Assessment of Electronic Fetal Monitoring." *Women and Health* 7(3&4):115-134.

Holmes, H. B.; Hoskins, B. & Gross, M. 1981a. *Birth Control and Controlling Birth, Women-Centered Perspectives*. Clifton, N.J.: Humana.

Holmes, H. B.; Hoskins, B. & Gross, M. 1981b. *The Custom-Made Child? Women-Centered Perspectives*. Clifton, N.J.: Humana.

Otten, A. 1985. "Women's Rights vs. Fetal Rights Looms as a Thorny and Divisive Issue." *Wall Street Journal*, April 12, 1985.

Parkes, Colin Murray and Weiss, Robert S. 1983. *Recovery from Bereavement*. Basic Books.

Patychuck, Dianne. 1985. "Ultrasound: The First Wave," *Healthsharing* (Fall 1985):25-28.

Rothman, B. K. 1986. *The Tentative Pregnancy*. New York: Viking.

Statmeyer, M. E. & Christman, C. L. 1982. "Biological Effects of Ultrasound" *Women and Health* 7(3&4):65-81.

Whitbeck, Caroline. 1984. "A Different Reality: Feminist Ontology." *Beyond Domination: New Perspectives on Women and Philosophy*. Edited by Carol C. Gould. Rowman & Allanheld.

Whitbeck, Caroline. 1983. "The Moral Implications of Regarding Women as People: New Perspectives on Pregnancy and Personhood." *Abortion and the Status of the Fetus*. Edited by W.B. Bondeson, H.T. Engelhardt, Jr., S.F. Spicker, and D. Winship. D. Reidel Pub. Co.

Whitbeck, Caroline. 1985. "Why the Attention to Paternalism in Medical Ethics?" *Journal of Health Politics, Policy and Law* 10(1):181-187.

Power, Certainty, and the Fear of Death

Rebecca Sarah

SUMMARY. Reproductive technology has been poorly used because both health care providers and clients unrealistically expect it to prevent all death and uncertainty. Because of this we often get the risks, side effects, and inaccurate information without benefits. Poorly used reproductive technology also deskills both providers and clients. Used realistically and controlled by women—birthing women and midwives—this technology can be of great benefit to us and our children.

The Shadow of Death

The shadow of death has always hung over the birthing bed.
Time was, every midwife was a baptiser.
Usually, safe passage, but every midwife could wrap a
    shroud

Many of these ideas were thought out in conversations with Trudy Cox, CNM, and with Myla Kabat-Zinn. I have benefited greatly from their wisdom and experience. Jessie Stickgold-Sarah lent me her word processor, and Bob Stickgold taught me how to use it with intelligence, humor, and patience. Talking with Dr. Ruth Perry helped me focus my thinking about how technology can deskill us. Patricia Cobb understands what midwifery is and reminds me when I lose sight of it. Bruce E. Martin, Sonographer, gave me useful technical information and examples from his experience. In other ways, Dr. Glenn Rothfeld helped me a great deal. I want to thank Janet Leigh and Joan Richards for helping me to give birth at home. Dr. Mitchell Levine taught me a lot, gave me unusual space and support in which to work, and set an example of sound medical decision making. I have learned a great deal from knowing and working with Michelle Harrison, Narinjan Khalsa, Cathleen Cooney, Trudy Cox, Myla Kabat-Zinn, Beth Shearer, Janet Leigh, and Judy Luce. Most of all, I want to thank my daughters, Jessie and Cory, for everything.

and walked a few times a year with the funeral
and wept with the mother. And went on.
The shadow of death still hangs over the birthing bed.
But now we have the arrogant frightened doctors,
striding in the halls with their loud voices,
the scurrying obedient nurses.
And every death is paid for
with anger, incredulity, fault, someone's fault, lawsuits,
and the mother weeps alone
and no one else is permitted to weep.

Reproductive technology is neither a savior nor a nemesis, neither the cause of all our problems nor the solution to them. I am a lay midwife and in over ten years of caring for childbearing women, I have known many people who believe it is one or the other. But I think that how this technology affects our lives now and in the future has much more to do with the expectations of both consumers and care providers, and with how decisions are made about the use of this technology, than with anything inherent in the technology.

None of the technology used to achieve pregnancy, to test and evaluate pregnancy, or to intervene in birth will save us from all of biology's inconveniences, errors, and tragedies. Nor can it guarantee us healthy babies, or pregnancy when and only when we want it. There are many reasons why we have come to expect perfection and close to total control over our bodies, and why doctors think they can provide this. I think it is this very expectation that leads to the misuse of technology and thereby to most of the problems with it.

Neither are these technologies simply a menace designed by male doctors and scientists to control women, as some women fear. Some men's unacknowledged deep desire to know and control what goes on in women's bodies is the source of certain of our troubles, but most reproductive technologies were originally invented for better reasons, in response to real human suffering and problems, and they can be of benefit to us at times.

Unrealistic expectations of reproductive technologies among some doctors, technicians and childbearing women are matched by unrealistic expectations of nature and women's bodies by others, including people in the feminist and women's health movement.

The natural childbirth movement and lay midwifery are based on the feminist idea that women's bodies work, that giving birth is a natural function of our bodies and not a medical problem. I believe in this idea even more now than I did ten years ago when, with a new baby and past years of political work in the women's movement and the New Left, I decided to become a lay midwife. Experience with high-intervention hospital births has made me even more aware of how powerfully well our bodies do work. It amazes me that we are able to give birth at all under the unnatural, obstructive conditions of modern obstetrics. However, I think we also have to recognize that nature, including women's bodies, does not always work perfectly. It is not a beneficent force guaranteeing whatever is convenient or safe for us. A certain amount of death and suffering are entirely natural.

Very few of us are really willing to do without reproductive technology entirely, but we needn't accept its routine and inappropriate use as the price of its rare but crucial benefits. By keeping control of birth in the hands of women, mainly birthing women and, secondarily, midwives, good decisions can be made about the times when technology can help us. At the same time, we can learn more about, and help each other believe in, our power to bring forth new life. No matter what technology becomes available, most babies will always be best and most safely born with their mothers standing or kneeling or squatting in their own bedrooms, surrounded by people who care for them, including a couple of experienced midwives. But the times it doesn't work like this can still belong to us (to all of us as a group of human beings trying to live together, and primarily to birthing women) if we have the power and knowledge to make the necessary decisions about testing and intervention, and if we make them knowing realistically that not *all* suffering can be prevented.

Mothering is a metaphor for all of this. Mostly we raise our children well, sometimes against great odds, better than any expert could tell us. But things don't always go well, and when they don't, there's not necessarily anyone at fault. There are times when we can use help, and the losses and failures, the tears and fears, are part of our mothering, too, not just the good days and birthday cakes and things that turn out as we plan.

As a childbirth educator or midwife in this culture it's easy to think of the many times we've seen unnecessary technological intervention in pregnancy and birth. But I got a letter recently that reminded me forcefully of the other side of this. It was from a group of midwives working in Nicaragua, describing conditions there and asking for money and supplies. They mentioned that they did not have pitocin, a hormone that stimulates contractions of the uterus and that is used to start or speed labor as well as to stop postpartum hemorrhage. A donation of $10.00 would buy a lot of pitocin. I was horrified at the idea of midwives having to practice without this drug, and immediately sent $10.00, although I am also horrified by the overuse of pitocin here, where it is most often given for the convenience of doctors or just to create the illusion of control over the labor. As a midwife and a childbirth educator, I've spent a lot of time explaining to women the alternatives to pitocin and the risks of using it. Yet the image of a midwife in another continent struggling to control a hemorrhage without pitocin stayed in my mind, and made me realize again that women do need access to medical technology too, as well as protection from it.

Ultrasound is another example of the double-edged nature of reproductive technology. There are a few situations where an ultrasound is clearly in the best interests of a pregnant women: where there is a problem or a suspected problem in pregnancy or birth and where more information can really help us make better decisions.

For example, one situation that comes to mind immediately where ultrasound is needed is a placenta previa, or suspected placenta previa. A previa is a case where the placenta has grown over, or too near, the cervix. If it covers the cervix, then of course the baby cannot be born vaginally and both mother and baby will bleed heavily, possibly fatally, in labor as the cervix starts to dilate. Caesarean section is clearly needed in this case and safest for both mother and baby. Generally there are warning signs of a placenta previa, but they are not always definitive. Painless vaginal bleeding in the last trimester virtually always accompanies a previa. But this kind of bleeding can happen for other, benign, reasons too. A woman with recurrent painless vaginal bleeding in late pregnancy needs to know where the placenta is, and so does the doctor or midwife taking care of her. This is something that only an ultrasound can show accurately.

When the uterus is much larger than expected for the length of the pregnancy, one possibility is that the woman is carrying twins. Another is that the pregnancy began earlier than thought and is further advanced. It is important to know which: we can give better care to a woman carrying twins if we know they are there. We can quite often tell the difference in other ways, but sometimes signs are contradictory, the woman may not remember her menstrual history or have very irregular cycles. In this case again, ultrasound is the most effective diagnostic tool.

"Dating" the pregnancy by ultrasound can be useful, too. We don't know precisely when the baby will be born and we don't need to know. But we can give better care if we know, when labor begins, whether the baby is premature or "postmature," or within the range of time when it's healthiest and most common to be born: 37 to 42 weeks. For example, most midwives agree that only babies coming between 37 and 42 weeks should be born at home. That means we need to know when 37-42 weeks *is*. In most pregnancies, we can be accurate about dates without ultrasound, using a careful history and a careful watch on the landmark events of early pregnancy that almost always occur at specific times. Occasionally these signs are insufficient or contradictory and an ultrasound in the first trimester can reveal when the baby was conceived. If we're too causal about dates early in pregnancy, and don't use ultrasound, we could end up transferring a woman to the hospital because our best estimate is that she's in premature labor when in fact she's on time and could safely birth at home. Conversely, we risk attending premature or postmature births at home; most home birth professionals agree that these babies should be born in the hospital.

Probably the first piece of medical technology to be widely adopted by midwives was the Doptone, an ultrasound device that can pick up the baby's heartbeat during labor. Using a Doptone, we can monitor the baby easily with the mother in any position. She can stand, squat to push, be on her hands and knees (a good position for pushing). With the fetoscope, a device similar to a stethoscope and a precursor to the Doptone, we cannot always hear well except if the mother lies down, a position that increases pain and slows labor. Monitoring then is actually less intrusive with the Doptone than with the fetoscope. The fetoscope is fine for early labor, but many home birth midwives use the Doptone in spite of worries about the long term effects of ultrasound because it allows the mother to labor more spontaneously and naturally in active and second stage labor.

Much of the reproductive technology available is aimed at problems of infertility. While there are certainly some risks to the infertility technology, both biomedical and social, and many cases of infertility which technology cannot help, there are also tremendous benefits for some women. The desire to have a baby is not simply a product of our conditioning; for some of us, it's one of the deepest desires we have, and a wanted pregnancy can be a great joy. Artificial insemination is a perfect example of a technology women, individual women, can control. For lesbian couples especially, AI may offer the only acceptable means of conceiving.

More complex technologies can also be of great benefit in some cases. Drugs that induce ovulation have medical and social problems, but I know several women who almost certainly never would have conceived without them and who now have much-loved children.

Cesarean section is probably the most resented and feared intervention in birth these days, for good reason. It has the most severe consequences: there are very significant health risks to a woman undergoing this major surgery, and the emotional experience is often devastating. In addition there are weeks of painful recovery and it is clear that the vast majority of cesarean sections done now are unnecessary. Yet this surgery is occasionally life-saving. A transverse baby, one who lies sideways across the uterus, cannot be born vaginally. A baby in severe distress can often be saved by prompt cesarean. In addition to being genuinely life-saving, the necessary cesarean is not a negative emotional experience. In my experience, a woman who trusts that her labor was interrupted for a very good reason is often disappointed but she doesn't usually experience the rage or deep sadness and sense of loss felt by the many women who know quite well that their surgery wasn't necessary.

Using reproductive technology for what it can't do well leads to most of the problems. Asking technology to answer questions it can't answer, or using it routinely to solve problems that aren't there or are extremely unlikely to be there, leads to two bad effects. One is the bad care given and sometimes damage done when we get wrong information from technology and persist in acting on it. The other is that poor use of unnecessary tests and procedures deskills us and undermines our strengths as practitioners and mothers. Machines have the capacity to make weaklings of us, or to extend our strength, depending on how we use them.

There are many examples of how tests inappropriately used give wrong information that practitioners persist in acting on. Every doctor or midwife that I discussed this with had an example to offer.

For example, Electronic Fetal Monitoring has often been used inappropriately. The monitor has never been proven to be of benefit for routine use on healthy women in normal labor. When it began to be used this way, usually by inexperienced staff uncertain how to interpret the tracings, there's much evidence that it tripled the cesarean rate without changing the percentage of healthy babies. That means that with monitors women have the same chance (very high) of giving birth to a healthy baby, but 3 times the rate of surgical deliveries. It also confines the woman to bed, usually on her back — the position that allows the machine to get a good tracing, which is also the most painful position for labor. Active labor in a supine position can even *cause* fetal distress due to impaired blood flow to the baby. Many studies show that skilled attendant with a fetoscope or Doptone can monitor a baby just as effectively as with Electronic Fetal Monitoring. Further, the monitor encourages the medical staff, the family, and sometimes the woman herself to focus on the machine rather than the woman and her work and her needs. Many times I have entered a labor room to find the bed pushed over against the wall with a frightened woman trying desperately to cope with her labor, while the residents and nurses and her husband cluster eagerly around the machine to see what was happening.

I mentioned previously the value of having an accurate due date. Ultrasound can do this well within certain limits. Using it for this purpose outside those limits is a perfect example of technology being used that gives wrong data that is then acted on. After 34 weeks, ultrasound is no help: it can't distinguish age from size at that stage. Everyone knows this — it's in all the texts. But a hunger for answers and certainty drives physicians to order ultrasound pictures when they suddenly doubt the dates in late pregnancy or when a woman comes for prenatal care for the first time late in her pregnancy. The problem with this is that, left to herself, the woman will probably give birth to a mature baby, that is, one born between 37 and 42 weeks. However if a due date is created by a machine, labor may be induced or even a cesarean section done on the assumption that the baby is very late. Some premature babies are born by elective cesarean section or following labor induced for assumed postmaturity. While there are sometimes other factors in decision making, often a wrong due date from a late ultrasound is a large part of the justification for intervention that hastens birth.

Similarly, when a woman has had years of 28 or 30 day menstrual cycles, it doesn't make sense to move the due date by a week because of an ultrasound reading, yet this is often done. The reports themselves say "plus or minus one week" and the technicians tell us the same. An ultrasound in the first half of pregnancy tells us accurately in what *month* the baby was conceived, within that month an accurate and consistent menstrual history is our best source of information. Yet I often see women whose due dates have been moved up a week because of an ultrasound. This doesn't matter except at the end, when intervention may be done on the basis of dates that were inaccurate to start with.

Using x rays of the mother's pelvis and the baby's head to determine whether there is enough room for the baby to fit through and be born vaginally is another example of misuse of technology. It may seem a sensible technological aid, but x rays are not predictive of either normal or complicated births. My friend Beth, a childbirth educator who often attends hospital births to provide support to the woman, tells of a client of hers who was laboring in a big teaching hospital where such x rays are relied on. The woman was "stuck" at about 8 or 9 centimeters and hadn't made progress for several hours. To most midwives and some obstetricians, there's nothing abnormal about this, but to her doctor it was troubling enough to order x rays. Luckily, it takes a while to take the films and to process them: enough time, in this case, for the woman to give birth.

She was nursing her new baby when the technician came back with films that showed "absolute disproportion," meaning that the baby's head was clearly and absolutely too big to fit through the mother's pelvis. This would be funny except that it happens over and over again — most midwives can tell of a case. I had a client myself whose first baby was born by cesarean because the x ray said there was no room, yet she gave birth vaginally to a baby two pounds larger a few years later. But women and babies continue to have useless radiation and surgery because doctors want a quick definite answer.

It can be very difficult to make decisions about when to use cesarean section to end a long labor when there's no progress or extremely slow progress. There are no absolute criteria, no way to be sure afterwards that one has made the right decision. Those of us who take care of women in labor have to learn to live with this kind of uncertainty.

Another bad effect of inappropriate reliance on technology is that it deskills midwives and medical practitioners, undermines us and causes us to lose complex clinical skills. It undermines us as mothers, too, in an analogous way to be discussed below.

One example of deskilling is the loss of the ability to use the fetoscope, a device like a stethoscope that allows us to hear the unborn baby's heartbeat. At times, the technological ways of monitoring a baby's heartbeat have their advantages, but now that they are being used routinely, many obstetrical offices no longer own a fetoscope and many labor and delivery nurses are not trained in their use. I think this is a mistake: the fetoscope is cheap, totally harmless, portable and can be used under any circumstances. Also, if we someday find out that there is a clear hazard in using ultrasound (used in both the EFM and the Doptone), we're not going to feel too bad about the times we used those devices when it was clearly beneficial or necessary. But we'll feel pretty silly about the times we did so just because it was more convenient or because no one knew anymore how to use a fetoscope.

More subtle skills can be lost, too. I had a client recently who showed some signs of IUGR (Intrauterine Growth Retardation). In the last 10 weeks of pregnancy, she stopped gaining weight, and her uterine size as measured abdominally did not increase at a stage when usually the baby is growing rapidly. Her diet was excellent and she was a small, light-boned person. I hadn't really expected a big baby—she didn't smoke or have high blood pressure, so it was rather unlikely she had IUGR. But I sent her for ultrasound, which indicated she was 3-4 weeks behind, enough to be worrisome. We all worried. The day I got the report, I also saw my client and carefully palpated the baby for size and position. I'll never forget the feel of that baby's head, or my thoughts: "I must be way off. This baby feels good sized to me." As it turned out I was right, there, and wrong in my assumption that the ultrasound necessarily knew more than I did. She gave birth a few days before her due date to a healthy eight-pound baby.

We tend to treat the ultrasound as an absolute arbiter rather than one more piece of information. It was appropriate to ask this client to have an ultrasound, and I'll use it again, but I'll never forget to use my hands and my head, too. Yet I see young doctors being trained to rely on the machine, never developing these other skills, not even knowing they exist. In another generation, will doctors have forgotten all this, and see the skills in midwives' hands, the ability to feel for size and position, to tell polyhydramnios (excess amniotic fluid) from twins, as a kind of witchery, mysterious and unreliable?

When one kind of medical intervention becomes the automatic solution to a difficult problem we lose our other skills and abilities. The growing practice of delivering by cesarean all first babies who are breech and many breeches born to mothers who have given birth before, is leading to the loss of two skills among our obstetricians. One is the ability to determine *which* breeches could safely be born vaginally. The other is how to deliver them. In another generation we may have to deliver all our breeches surgically, because there will be no one who knows how to do any differently. It may take less time than that, if young doctors are taught nothing about this, and experienced ones are pressured into setting those skills aside in favor of automatic surgery.

There's a final, and more pernicious, problem. I know at least one obstetrician who sends *every* pregnant woman for three ultrasounds in early pregnancy, to "foster bonding." Many others, and some Certified Nurse Midwives, do the same in response to the first sign of anxiety or ambivalence on a pregnant woman's part. Far from "fostering bonding" I think this interferes with and undermines the complex, subtle, and powerful ways we experience pregnancy and thereby prepare to love and care for our children.

What goes on in a pregnant woman as she accepts the pregnancy, imagines and begins to believe in, and then to love, the baby, may look fragile and unpredictable. But it is a powerful and trustworthy process; it is the foundation of the strongest bond between human beings, and the basis for all the others: the love between mother and child. This natural process does involve anxiety, ambivalence, fear, and sometimes painful self-discovery. If practitioners can't bear to be confronted by these uncomfortable feelings, they may think they can use the machine to say unarguably, "There, SEE, that's your baby, you are a mother, everything is fine." Doing this is a discounting and loss of the midwifery skill of listening, understanding, empathizing, reassuring . . . helping the woman deal with her feelings, and move through this stage of life: helping her grow.

Worse, by teaching the woman to look to authority figures and machines for simple answers to the dilemmas and hard times of mothering, we teach her not to explore her own inner resources, her family and community, her own instinctive and hormonal responses to the baby. It is these that do in fact make mothers of us and if as a culture we decide to override and ignore these strengths we weaken our capacity for human connection and love.

The times when reproductive technology is to our advantage have been discussed above: when there is a known problem or a reasonable likelihood of a problem, and when information that can contribute to better decisions is available only, or optimally, through technology. These are obvious criteria and no one disagrees with them. Why then do we consistently, practitioners and consumers alike, demand more of technology than it can give us, especially when there is clearly a cost to doing so? Some testing and intervention are done to protect the doctor "medicolegally," but that doesn't account for most of it.

I think it is largely our fear of death and uncertainty. No one, in any time or place, wants to face the inevitability of pain, loss, and death. Loss of our children, or damage to them is particularly unbearable. And childbearing women are generally young and healthy, at a stage of life when people feel, and are seen, as safe from health problems. So the idea of risk, and possible death (however unlikely) is hard to take. There are many ways that life in America in the 80s protects most of us from thinking about these things. Much has been written elsewhere about how insulated from death — and birth — most of us are. What we call science has given us so much — we'd like to believe it could give us absolute safety, too, and absolute certainty about what's going on in the body and what to do about it.

Those who reject too much technology in favor of a more "natural" approach to their own health and that of their babies and children tend to ascribe to nature the same benevolent power to protect us from all pain and loss. In the natural childbirth and holistic health movements, homilies like "birth is a natural event, not a disease" and "the body's own healing powers" imply that if we do everything right the body will work perfectly, we will never have serious unsolvable health problems, and woman's power to bring new life into the world will never bring death or imperfection.

This is not really so different from what doctors are taught: it's never said, but especially the most caring doctors seem to come out believing that if they are careful enough, and up to date enough, there will never be a "preventable" death. They can accept deaths on the frontiers of knowledge; it's sad, but not unexpected when tiny premature babies die. But the mature baby of a healthy mother? They should never die, and the idea that a mother could die is, deep down, totally unacceptable.

I'm not suggesting we should be sanguine or too accepting of these deaths, or any deaths. Horror and grief and an effort to do everything we can to prevent them are appropriate reactions. But there will always, at least in the foreseeable future, be some deaths, and many problems we can't solve, situations without clearcut answers. Rather than ordering a test or procedure anyway, to convince ourselves and our clients that we *do* know, or that we are "doing everything" to help a woman conceive or a pregnancy to continue safely, midwives and doctors must be able to say, "I don't know," and women and their families must be able to hear it. One obstetrician I know has been very careful lately, to say, "I don't know," when that's the case and he's noticed that some clients cannot accept it. They persist in asking him to look it up, consult another doctor, and simply cannot hear that he's already done those things and *no one* knows. In this case, it is the patient's attitude that is a ticket to unnecessary and inappropriate use of technology.

Giving up the illusion that technology offers certainty and perfect safety means we let into our professional lives a lot of painful emotions. It means being willing to share the sadness and rage of a woman who will never be able to bear a child and to experience the grief of a family facing death. Because our training is different, it may be a little easier for midwives, lay midwives at least, to learn this, but it's hard for everyone. But if we can be at peace with these painful parts of our jobs, we will be able to stop demanding certainty, and perfect knowledge from technology. We'll use it, and our knowledge and experience, and the skills in our hands, each for what it can do, to give the best care we can.

A Short Answer to "Who Decides?"

William Ruddick

SUMMARY. Technology increases the control which experts and the medical professions exercise over conception, pregnancy, and childbirth. However, it is women and women alone who should make the ultimate decisions regarding their own childbearing.

Whatever the moral and metaphysical complexities of reproductive decisions, the answer to "Who should decide?" is clear. Women, and only women, should make decisions about their own childbearing. This does *not* exclude the concerns of men they care for, or the advice of men they trust. But it does exclude men, publicly or privately from having a veto or decisive voice in questions about the number, timing, or aborting of pregnancies, or the method of conception—or, the question of adoption versus conception.

My reasons are, roughly and simply, these: women bear children, and, for the most part they are responsible for their care. Either reason is, I think, sufficient to give a woman the sole right of decision; together, these reasons are conclusive. Nothing about the new means of conception and impregnation inclines me to qualify my view. On the contrary, these new techniques make assertion of a woman's rights of decision all the more important. Thanks to Ruth Hubbard (1984), Barbara Katz Rothman (1986) and others, we are becoming aware of technocratic pressures on conception, pregnancy, and childbirth. These pressures merely increase the control which experts and professions already exercise over women's reproduction. (Physicians prescribe or fit contraceptives; monitor diet

73

and weight gain during pregnancy; determine the method and time of delivery; allow or proscribe further pregnancies; and so forth.)

Let me note here two common sources of professional pressure:

(1) By way of inspiring themselves and justifying their privileges, members of professions proclaim dedication to general human goods: physicians, to promoting Life and Health; lawyers, to Justice and Order; soldiers, to National Security and Honor; the clergy, to Morality and Salvation. More specifically (modern) physicians speak of their professional commitment to Respecting and Prolonging Life. But note: by so doing, they render abortion and infant euthanasia professionally suspect. Likewise, these abstract goals make medically assisted conception and fetal therapy immediately commendable. Physicians moved by these professional abstractions will accordingly present *in vitro* fertilization (IVF), abortion, or fetal therapy in ways appropriately colored by these general goals. Fetal surgeons, for example, may tendentiously state a woman's options so: "You could abort the child, or we could increase its chances of survival by implanting a shunt."

(2) When professional abstractions are powered by professional optimism, pressure on patients is even greater. Thus, without talk of "chances of survival," fetal surgeons may say simply, "You could abort the baby, or we can save it by implanting a shunt." Optimists typically disregard probabilities of success, low or high; they are moved rather by *possibilities*, confident in their capacities to beat the odds. (Optimists see the glass as half full because they assume that they can easily fill it, or, at least, that they can find ways to make do with only half.)

Optimists are not irrational. In novel undertakings, there are no firm probability estimates either to ignore or to take seriously. Hence optimism may seem fully justified by its moral benefits: optimistic professionals induce hope, enthusiasm, and compliance from their associates and clients. On the other hand, physicians' optimism may produce careless underestimation of risks and costs. Thus, women eager to have children may be misled by professional optimism to undergo invasive procedures with little chance of success. The resulting failures may surprise and sadden both physician and patient. But at least the physician has the consolation of acquiring new data for the medical profession's "war on sterility." For

the woman, however, there may be no comparable, abstract consolation, but only the deeper disappointment in a particular life she
finds unsatisfactory without children.

If "let women decide" is to be more than a liberal slogan, then
professional men (and women) must identify and restrain the ways
in which professional abstractions and optimism subtly limit or distort the options they present to women. There are several obvious
measures. First, physicians might give more thought to concrete
lives in their diverse particularity and less to Life and Quality of
Life. For example, women's varied accounts of pregnancy could
become part of obstetrical texts and training, in place of general
descriptions of The Pregnant Woman. Secondly, professionals
might allow and encourage women to speak freely about ambivalent
feelings and second thoughts about their medical treatment. Patron-
izing impatience, in the name of efficiency, could be seen to reflect
sexist attitudes. And, thirdly, physicians might collaborate with
other professionals (e.g., midwives), and thereby mitigate the iso-
lating, alienating impact of high medical technology on conception,
pregnancy and childbirth.

Each of these measures runs counter to paternalistic tradition,
and patriarchal ideology of which paternalism is part. Patriarchy (as
the name bears witness) presupposes a father's control over children, as well as over the reproductive decisions by which they are
generated. Such control was rationalized by familiar assumptions
about women's needs, desires, capacities, physiology, as well as
dicta about the importance and composition of families. Whether
control of children or, as now claimed, control of women is the
primary patriarchal motive, it is obvious that children play an important part in men's lives, in our choices of work and pleasures, in
our sense of self. This is so even for men who do not need children
to assist them in their work, or men who do not worry about traditional proofs of virility, or the continuance beyond death of their
name, their lineage, their genes, or their projects. Ironically, even
feminist men, learning the pleasures of childcare, may unwittingly
add to traditional reproductive pressures on women and reject the
simple exclusionary answer I proposed at the outset.

Not all objections to women as sole deciders are either professional or patriarchal. For example, women who decide to employ or

to act as maternal surrogates are criticized as engaging in an exploitative, commercial transaction. Some critics call for a legal ban on this "baby selling and buying" (Holder 1984). But why, in a culture which "commodifies" and commercializes most work and many human relations, should reproduction be singled out (along with sex) for legal stigma? Why are women — especially poor, untrained women — to be denied a familiar form of labor which they may prefer to the other exploitative options they have? (Some women defend surrogacy on the grounds that it is work within the home, work which allows them to spend more time with their own children than any alternative they have.) Rather than preventing women from choosing this form of work, the law might attempt to protect such choices from the coercive pressures women, especially poor women, suffer in the work world. Before acting on professional (and perhaps classest) assumptions of what is good for women and children, legal professionals should attend carefully to women's accounts of these arrangements. Otherwise, in pursuit of abstract ideals, professionals may enact legislation which, as so often, falls most heavily on those already oppressed by the conditions of their lives.

REFERENCES

Holder, A. 1984. "Surrogate Motherhood: Babies for Fun and Profit." *Law, Medicine, & Health Care* 12:115.

Hubbard, R. 1984. "Personal Courage is Not Enough: Some Hazards of Childbearing in the 1980s." Pp. 331-355 in *Test-Tube Women*, edited by Rita Arditti, Renate Duelli Klein, & Shelley Minden. Boston: Pandora Press.

Rothman, B. K. 1986. *The Tentative Pregnancy: Prenatal Diagnosis and the Future of Motherhood*. New York: Viking.

What the King
Can Not See

Gena Corea

SUMMARY. This paper contrasts the ways in which the physician-scientist developing *in vitro* fertilization ("the king") sees the world and the way women experience it. It challenges the truth of what the king sees: i.e., that women have a desperate will to be mothers that must be fulfilled at all costs; that the way to make infertile women mothers is through the use of new reproductive technologies; that IVF programs are quite successful and that women who enter these programs actually come away with babies.

I am interested in unreality. That is, women's experience. Women's perceptions. But I will talk to you about reality as well. The reality of such new reproductive technologies as *in vitro* fertilization. The philosopher Marilyn Frye (1983) has written an essay on the politics of reality in which she states:

Reality is that which is.
The English world "real" stems from a word which meant
  regal, of or pertaining to the king.
'Real" in Spanish means royal.
Real property is that which is proper to the king.
Real estate is the estate of the king.
Reality is that which pertains to the one in power, is that
  over which he has power, is his domain, his estate, is
  per to him.
The ideal king reigns over everything as far as the eye can
  see. His eye. What he cannot see is not royal, not real.

He sees what is proper to him.
To be real is to be visible to the king . . .

Reality is that which pertains to the one in power, and in the context in which I am writing today, the one in power is the physician-scientist engaged in reproductive technology, or, collectively, what I call the pharmacracy — a power elite of physicians who exercise social control through medicine. The pharmacracy — that is the king.

And what can the king see? It is important to know this because whatever the king can see is real. But for women, it is even more important to know what the king can not see.

The king can see that women have a desperate will to be mothers. This is a natural desire which must be fulfilled at all costs. The way to make infertile women mothers is through use of the new reproductive technologies. Indeed, these women flock to physicians pleading with them to develop new technologies so they can experience a serene and joyful motherhood. They enter the IVF programs, get their babies (for IVF is quite successful), hold them happily and say, "It's a miracle. I'm so happy and so grateful to my doctors."

This is what the king can see. This is reality as presented by physicians and disseminated to all of us through the media.

Let me name these points again one by one and talk as well about what the king can not see.

Women have a desperate will to be mothers. What the king can not see here are the social forces constructing a woman's "will" to be a mother. I am not saying that there is no such thing as a desire for a child unstructured by the society in which we live. And I acknowledge that both men and women share some common motives for wanting children.[1] But there are added forces shaping a woman's will to be a mother, forces which do not act on men.

How is a woman's will to be a mother structured?

1. By fixing a woman's function as reproductive and sexual. The fixing is done through the apparatuses of civil society. When I say "civil society," I'm referring to a distinction made by the Italian philosopher Antonio Gramsci (cited in Graebner 1984). He divided politics into two areas. The first was "political society" consisting of public institutions like the courts, police, army, the electoral pro-

cess. The second was "civil society" including schools, churches, and the popular press.

Gramsci considered the civil society the most important apparatus the ruling class has for controlling the people. It uses this apparatus for securing and maintaining the "consent" of the governed.

I want to take some insights William Graebner has concerning "civil society" and apply them to the situation of women "choosing" to enter IVF programs or to become surrogate mothers (Graebner 1984). All cultures, totalitarian or democratic, have mechanisms of social engineering that accomplish the task of getting women to perform the functions — sexual and reproductive — it sets for them. Various societies do this with more or less force. Our democratic societies do it through a hegemonic process called "freedom of choice."

There is a very extensive literature documenting the ways in which civil society — schools, churches, media, medicine, language — structure the choices of girls and women.[2] They repeatedly beep out the message: "Women are for bearing babies. Bearing babies is woman's function in life. Women are for sex. Being sexy for men is woman's function in life." When a woman's identity is largely stripped down to the two functions civil society says she has — reproductive and sexual — she tends to internalize that valuation of herself. The work civil society does in stripping woman's identity down to only two of many possible components helps shape her "desperate" will to be a mother.

How is a woman's will be to be a mother structured?

2. By a manipulation of her emotions and motivations. The propaganda that if a woman is infertile, she loses her most basic identity as a woman, has a coercive power. Emotional coercion can be as powerful as physical coercion. Once woman's prime function has been fixed as reproductive, a "barren" woman who cannot fulfill that function is threatened with abandonment, isolation, loss of love, rejection from the family group, social humiliation. All these are the symbolic equivalents of death. When her husband or her doctor, in discussing her infertility, appeals to her unconscious fears of abandonment, then this manipulation of her emotions helps structure her will to become a mother.

The doctor's authority stands behind the notion that it is quite reasonable for a woman to go through any torture in order to fulfill her "natural" role and bear a baby. In a submission to the Warnock Commission on reproductive technology in Britain, after describing the considerable social pressure on women to be mothers, the group "Women in Medicine" stated: "Medical opinion too exerts a pressure on women: the high status of doctors in our society gives them authority and indeed power. If a doctor thinks it reasonable for women to go to any lengths in order to bear a child, women will be confirmed in their suspicion that motherhood is a goal to be pursued at all costs" (Women in Medicine 1984).

How is a woman's will to be a mother structured?

3. By withholding from her vital information about the meaning of motherhood. The socially validated meaning of motherhood is that of rosy feminine fulfillment. Now it is true that many women feel, through motherhood, a deeper love than they have ever known. Some — not all — find motherhood a powerful experience. But they also find it frustrating, boring, exhausting, draining. Some women stagger through motherhood on high doses of tranquilizers. But women's negative experiences of motherhood are not incorporated into the official version of "reality" (Spender 1980). They are not what the king can see. They are only what women see, so they are, by definition, not real.

How is a woman's will to be a mother structured?

4. By the social devaluation of women's labor and skills, which pressures women into motherhood (Rothman 1985). Women are largely confined to low-paying service jobs and, in the United States, earn 59 cents to a man's dollar. By limiting women's job opportunities and pay and structuring society so that marriage is by and large a woman's livelihood, infertility becomes to a woman, among many other things, a threat to her livelihood. It threatens her survival.

5. The social devaluation of women's creativity and intelligence also pressures a woman into motherhood (Rothman 1985). While a woman who wants to pursue a career in physics or philosophy or deep-sea exploration may be lucky and encounter some individuals who will support her, she will get little encouragement from the apparatuses of civil society.

6. The social complacency about male violence and abuse towards women which reinforces women's lack of self-worth is another force structuring women's choices. Under that violence, I include rape, incest, woman-battery. Pornography, in eroticizing dominance and submission (that is, in making inequality sexy) also undermines women's sense of self-worth (Dworkin 1981).

As the sociologist Barbara Katz Rothman has written: "Lacking economic power, physical and emotional safety, women can be coerced into motherhood, which seems to offer a power-base from which to negotiate for some degree of status and protection" (Rothman 1985).

So the king sees that women have a will to be mothers. Which women? White women? Women of certain classes in developed countries like West Germany, Britain, the United States?

What about a woman in Bangladesh who has a will to be a mother? Her desire for motherhood will not prevent the local "motivator" from inducing her to be sterilized by offering her a sari and money desperately needed for food. The sterilizations are conducted in camps where, according to an investigation by an international committee, surgical gloves are often not even changed between operations (Hartmann 1987). Some women in Nepal who have a will to be mothers will also end up in sterilization camps where they are often given 5 to 10 milligrams of Valium as their only anesthesia.

The prevalence of infertility in some regions of the Third World is high. This is particularly so in Africa where in some areas 40% of all women have never borne a child by age 45, due to the high incidence of venereal disease (Bruce and Schearer 1983). But the king does not talk about the need for IVF programs in the Third World. He tends to talk rather about the so-called "population problem" there and the need for effective contraceptives like Depo-Provera and anti-pregnancy vaccines and campaigns to convince women to undergo sterilization.

The diaphram used with jelly or cream and spermicidal foams and suppositories used alone, appear to offer protection against some types of venereal disease. So, if the king is so concerned about the will of women to be mothers, why isn't he promoting use of barrier methods of contraception in the Third World — the only contraceptives to offer some protection against agents associated with venereal disease?

Two mavericks in the population control establishment, Judith Bruce and S. Bruce Schearer, write that " . . . in settings with high incidences of infertility, proper use of the condom and, possibly, of other barrier methods, can reduce the incidence of gonorrhea which is the primary cause of the infertility" (Bruce and Schearer 1983).

Yet, an average in 14 Third World countries surveyed by the World Fertility Survey, only 1.1% of all married contraceptive users used female barrier contraceptives. Bruce and Schearer attribute this at least partly to the failure of health delivery personnel to support, promote, and actively make these methods available to the people, while at the same time, they give "positive attention" to the Pill, IUDs, injectable contraceptives like Depo-Provera, and sterilization.

So the king is promoting use of the new reproductive technologies for infertile women in the West while, in the Third World, he is promoting contraceptives which provide no protection against fertility-destroying diseases, contraceptives which may indeed contribute to subsequent sterility.

If the "wrong" women have a will to be mothers, does the king see this? No. And if the king does not see it, it is not real.

As Barbara Rothman points out, women are socially rewarded for certain choices (for example, the choice to bear a child) and punished for others, and the rewards and punishments are handed out along race and class lines. In the United States, black women and poor white women who choose to bear children, who have a will to be mothers, and who at some point receive public assistance, are punished with social contempt, harassment, poverty. But all the organs of civil society go into action generating sympathy for white heterosexual married women who have a will to be mothers.

The king sees, not only that women (*some* women, *white* women, *married* women) have a will to be mothers, but that the way to make infertile women mothers is through the use of such technologies as *in vitro* fertilization.

What the king chooses not to see is the way in which many of these women became infertile in the first place.

In a magazine for ob/gyns, Dr. William R. Keye, who studied the causes of infertility presented by women at the University of Utah Medical Center, wrote: "We may cause more infertility than we care to believe." The experience at that center, he wrote: "suggests that iatrogenic [i.e., doctor-caused] infertility is common" (Keye 1982).

Physicians have caused a great deal of infertility through excessive surgery, and through the insertion, on a massive scale, of IUDs into women, and through experimentation on women with the drug diethylstilbestrol (DES).

When physicians are diagnosing pelvic pain, doing an infertility work-up, handling certain obstetric problems, or otherwise treating women, they sometimes use procedures which can impair the woman's fertility. Among these procedures are: cervical conization; dilation and curettage; endometrial biopsy; myomectomy; tubal insufflation; oophorectomy; cesarean section; hystereosalpingography; uterine suspension; hysteroscopy and hydropertubation (Keye 1982).

The IUD can also impair fertility by bringing on pelvic inflammatory disease (PID) which sometimes damages the reproductive organs. The risk of contracting PID is four to nine times higher in women with an IUD than in those without it (Keye 1982). This fact should come as no surprise: from its earliest days, the IUD went hand-in-hand with infection. In the 1930s and 1940s, the devices were associated with such a high rate of infection and other complications that the medical community abandoned them. Nothing changed to make them safer. But in the early 1960s, as fear of a "population explosion" spread, population control groups fixed on the discredited IUD as one device which could bring the birth rate down. These groups declared that "new data" showed how safe IUDs were. The "new data" consisted of two studies which, in fact, added nothing to the existent knowledge of the IUD. The author of one of the papers asserted that in his study, the IUD proved to be 25 times as safe as the diaphragm, an assertion any physician today would find laughable (Oppenheimer 1959). Nonetheless, population control groups, using that study, convinced physicians of the IUD's safety. Physicians began inserting the devices on a mass scale.

Many women into whom they were inserted became infertile. But this is not a tragedy. At least some find it easy to accept. At the first International Conference on Intra-uterine Contraception, sponsored by the Population Council in New York City in 1962, Dr. J. Robert Willson stated: "They [IUDs] are horrible things, they produce infection, they are outmoded and not worth using . . . but suppose one does develop an intrauterine infection and suppose she does end up with a hysterectomy and bilateral salpingo-oophorectomy? How serious is that for the particular patient and for the population of the world in general? Not very . . . Perhaps the individual patient is expendable in the general scheme of things, particularly if the infection she acquires is sterilizing but not lethal" (Quoted in Hartmann 1987).

Another cause of infertility is DES, the synthetic hormone. Despite the fact that there has never been any clear evidence that DES could prevent miscarriage, physicians gave the drug to women in the United States from the 1940s through the 1970s for that purpose. DES has since been associated with impaired fertility in daughters born to those women. They have a high incidence of upper genital tract abnormalities and impaired reproductive outcomes, investigators have found. Reliable data suggests that these daughters have an increased risk of ectopic pregnancies. Such pregnancies could damage the woman's oviducts, thus making her a candidate for more intervention: *in vitro* fertilization.

In July 1984, one IVF clinic reported on its experience with 20 DES daughters. Two of these women were victims, not only of DES, but of the IUD as well. They had tubal disease due to PID associated with prior use of that contraceptive (Musaher, Garcia and Jones 1984). So, after being injured by experimentation with the IUD and DES, they go on for more experimentation with the "repair" technology of IVF.

Physician attitudes toward women can also be a threat to our fertility. As Judy Norsigian, co-author of *Our Bodies, Ourselves*, charged at a government-sponsored seminar, the physician often lacks interest in and/or knowledge about prevention and treatment of diseases which can impair fertility. She said: "All too often, signs of inflammation and infection [indicating pelvic inflammatory disease] are either ignored or overlooked, even when a woman herself might point out the important symptoms. Sometimes these symptoms are passed off as psychosomatic'' (Wiesner 1979).

Male physicians too frequently dismiss women's complaints as products of neurotic imaginations, a problem I have documented at length in my first book (Corea 1985a).

The king does not see this. It is not real. He sees the benevolence of the pharmacracy which provides IVF treatment for desperate infertile women, but he does not see that the pharmacracy often helped destroy the women's fertility in the first place.

Nor does the king see the physical, emotional and spiritual damage these invasive procedures inflict on women. The women who are candidates for IVF have generally already been through an immense amount of medical probing and prodding, much of it painful and humiliating: endometrial biopsies, tubal insufflation (the filling of oviducts with pressurized carbon dioxide to see if the tubes are open); injecting dye into the uterus and oviducts, drug treatments, "blowing out" the tubes to maintain an opening; surgery, including laparoscopy.

Once in an IVF program, the manipulations of a woman's body and emotions begin in earnest: drugs administered; blood samples taken and hormones within measured; sometimes closing the oviducts using high· frequency electric current; ultrasound exams to estimate when women will ovulate; instilling sterile normal saline into a woman's bladder through a catheter for the ultrasound right before laparoscopy; laparoscopy for "egg capture," often repeated a number of times; sick, drowsy and sore from the operation she has just had, the woman is sometimes asked to arouse her husband sexually so he can masturbate for the sperm sample; transfer of an embryo into a woman's body during which cannula may traumatize the uterus.[2]

We need to hear from women how they experience all this. Certainly the king has not asked the women. We do, however, have some bits of information. In Australia, Dr. Barbara A. Burton, an IVF "patient," interviewed at length 12 women in an IVF support group who had been treated in six different IVF programs. She published her preliminary study. Some of the women's statements:

It [the IVF treatment] is embarrassing. You leave your pride
on the hospital door when you walk in and pick it up when you
leave. You feel like a piece of meat in a meat-works. But if
you want a baby badly enough you'll do it. (Burton 1985)

Burton quotes from an article on infertility: "In order to tolerate
the bodily invasion involved in investigations and treatment for infertility people may emotionally separate their minds and bodies."
The article then goes on to discuss this in terms of sexuality, stating
that under the pressure of treatment, it can be difficult for people to
feel "connected" enough to their own bodies to want to go on
making love with their partners.

But I would raise another question here. What kind of spiritual
damage does it do to women when they emotionally separate their
minds and bodies? Why does the king not see this as an issue of
some importance? We have heard some prostitutes say that during
intercourse with strangers who have rented the use of their bodies,
they too separate their minds from their bodies as a means of self-
protection. We have heard some people with multiple personalities
say that during extreme sexual abuse and torture in childhood, they
split off into separate personalities in order to make what was happening to them endurable. In order to survive.

What does it do to women in IVF "treatment" programs when,
to varying extents, they separate their minds and bodies in order to
make all the poking and prodding and embarrassments endurable? I
do not know the answer. But I want to know why, in the public
discussion of IVF, this is not even a question.

During the course of all these bodily manipulations, the woman
is on an emotional roller coaster. There is a cycle of hopes raised
and dashed which harms women in ways the king has not bothered
to examine. Let me describe some of the possible highs and lows on
that roller coaster:

The woman is accepted into the program. (A high.) But then,
after the expensive hormone treatment, no eggs grow to a size sufficient for "harvesting." (A low.) Or the eggs do ripen (a high) but
the doctors miscalculate the timing and the eggs ovulate and are
"lost" before they can get them. (A low.) Or the eggs ripen, but the
doctors can't get them out at laparoscopy. Or they got an egg but

it's abnormal. Or they got an egg but the husband can't masturbate in the stressful hospital conditions and so it is not fertilized. Or they got the egg (high), he got a sperm sample (high), but the egg is not fertilized (low). Or they got a fertilized egg but it doesn't implant. Or it implants but then, after several weeks, the woman miscarries. Or it remains implanted but it's ectopic. (A low, a devastating low.) Surgery is performed to remove the embryo.

The vast majority of women who go through IVF programs do not come away with a baby. The women Burton interviewed described the depression and grieving they experienced at failed IVF attempts. One women told her: "I just wanted to sit in a corner and die, but life goes on. There are beds to make and meals to cook."

All the women Burton interviewed wanted to know why their IVF attempts had not worked. They expressed a need for follow-up and a medical review after a failed treatment cycle, a need which was not met. One woman told her: "You don't get any feedback. It would be nice to be given a reason—a follow up phone call from the coordinator. It should be medical. You want to be told it's not your fault you bombed out. You just go home and feel a failure."

In addition to the poking and prodding involved in IVF treatment, women are also injected with powerful hormones. Some women are worried about what those hormones are doing to them. One woman told Burton:

> The professor tells us that according to the labels and his books they [the hormones] don't have side effects. Once someone comes out and is brave enough to say you get side effects, other women say so too. I think that's what he's worried about—that side effects are catching.

Most women Burton interviewed felt that they had not been given enough information about their treatment, that the IVF teams did not have the time necessary to talk to the women and explain what was happening. Most of the women, Burton reported, felt unable to ask questions as they saw the staff as being too busy. They were reluctant to jeopardize their treatment by being seen as "making waves" or being "pushy."

One woman told Burton: "I'd like the doctors to participate

more. They just pick up the eggs and put them back. The rest of the time you never see them. It's rush, rush, all the time. You don't like to ask questions. Even when they inform you, you don't take it all in. You don't like to phone them and make a nuisance."

Reality is very different for the physicians rushing around picking up eggs and putting them back in and for the women from whom the eggs are taken, back into whom they are put. The innumerable manipulations of a woman's body and the humiliation, as well as the pain involved in these procedures, threaten her well-being. The king does not see this. But Julie Melrose does. She is a woman who has been through a lot of surgery and thought and felt deeply about this issue. She wrote:

> There is a discrepancy between the way the doctor defines a surgical procedure and the way the person experiences it. Doctors have a tendency to look at surgical procedures in a technical and mechanical way. If they see a way that they can manipulate the body to accomplish what they want without posing an extremely high risk, they define the procedure as a piece of cake. From their position as mechanics, it *is* a piece of cake, that is, an easy procedure for them to perform.
>
> My feeling is that the human body has an integrity of its own and that it can not be violated, even in a way that the doctor may see as minor, without there being physical and emotional consequences for the person on whom the surgery is performed.
>
> Women often believe doctors when they say something is a piece of cake and believe that they shouldn't make a big deal about it but then, during and after the procedure, they often feel that it *was* a big deal and it did not feel like a piece of cake to *them*. Their immediate, and often lingering, response to the procedure in fact has depth and has strong emotions connected with it and may have changed them in significant ways." (Quoted in Corea 1985b)

Such new reproductive technologies as *in vitro* fertilization damage women in yet another way which the king does not recognize. Jalna Hanmer, the sociologist does. She points out that the implied message of the media and pharmacracy is that technology is best and can do the job of reproduction better than women can on their own. (For example, Prof. Carl Wood, head of an IVF team in Australia, announced last year that a study had found that children produced through IVF were brighter and better adjusted socially than children normally conceived.) The message is that men, through their technology, can perfect embryos and ensure perfect pregnancies, deliveries and babies. Women can not. This message, Hanmer writes, tears at female consciousness and identity. The new reproductive technologies remove the last woman-centered process from us.

After conversations with Hanmer, this is my interpretation of her theory:

Through the use of the new reproductive technologies, women's reproduction is now being obejectified in the same way woman's sexuality has been for centuries. Our sexuality has been so removed from ourselves and so male-defined for so long, that we really don't know what we mean when we say "woman-defined sexuality." We have no feel for it. We are too deeply divorced from our sexuality to be able to imagine a self-defined form of it. We do not feel, deep down, that our sexuality belongs to us. It belongs to men.

In contrast, this generation of women strongly feels that our reproductive capacity *does* belong to us. The women born today will not. Certainly the women born in 2050 will not. They will be divorced from their own procreative power as we are divorced from our sexuality. They will feel inadequate to reproduce. They will not believe they have the capacity to do so.

These will be women who, from their earliest days, grew up with the reality of IVF, embryo transfer, surrogate motherhood, artificial wombs, and sex predetermination technology. They will be women who have never known a world without "superovulation" and "ovum capture." From childhood, these women will have watched television news reports involving the "Storage Authority," that is, the board in charge of frozen sperm, eggs and human embryos.

They will be women whose own "mothers" may have supplied the egg from which they were generated, *or* the uterus in which they were gestated, or perhaps neither. These women of 2050 will know that among women, there are egg donors and there are breeders or gestators and there are those who provide various body parts and fluids used in reproduction (for example, urine from which hormones are extracted for use in superovulating the ovaries of younger females). But no one woman procreates a baby all by herself. This will be so because (as I have discussed elsewhere) by 2050, use of the new reproductive technologies will have expanded beyond the original category of women — the infertile — for whom it was first touted.

This, then, might be the reproductive consciousness of our daughters in the 21st century: "Reproduction is a complicated intellectual and technical feat performed by teams of highly skilled men who use, as raw material for their achievements, the body parts of a variety of interchangeable females."

The autonomous ability of these women to control their procreative processes is diminished. *Another* aspect of a woman's self-definition is undermined which, when added to her loss of political, economic and social power, transforms her consciousness of herself as an inferior being. She feels even more inferior to men than women today believe themselves to be.

Loss of autonomous reproduction is one more fundamental layer leading to a loss of Self.

This loss is not visible to the king. You will never hear him speak of it.

And finally, the king sees that *in vitro* fertilization is quite successful.

He does not see that IVF only looks "successful" when the definition of what constitutes "success" is controlled by those with a stake in appearing successful. This became apparent to Susan Ince and myself when we conducted a survey of the 108 IVF clinics in the United States in 1985. Ince was then articles editor of *The Medical Tribune*, a newspaper for physicians, and we conducted the survey for the *Tribune* (Corea and Ince, 1985, July 3). Half (54) the clinics responded to our five-page mail questionnaire. Each was operational and collecting fees ranging from $1,375 to $7,000 and averaging $4,085 per IVF attempt.

We found that half the responding clinics have *never* sent a woman home with a baby. Of the 26 clinics which did have babies,

20 had five or fewer. Yet many of these clinics claim astonishing success rates. For example, one university-affiliated clinic has produced no IVF babies but, according to its calculation, has a success rate of 18.2%. A private clinic on the West Coast has no IVF babies but its success is 22%. The IVF Program at a major medical school reported no babies and a success rate of 25%.

The questionnaire allowed clinic directors to enter their success rate and how it is calculated. We found that there is no uniform definition of "success." A clinic can define success however it likes and no one calls it to account. On our questionnaires, many chose "percentage of pregnancies per laparoscopy" as the measure of success. But the fact that there are pregnancies does not mean that there will actually be births. Some of the pregnancies are chemical—that is, simply slight elevations in the level of hormones produced during pregnancy (HCG). And many clinics count as IVF "successes" miscarriages and ectopic pregnancies, which also will not lead to live births.

I'm going to list some facts that I do not think the king would dispute. And these facts mean that there is a Reproduction Revolution underway:

1. Throughout the industrialized world, human embryos are now being created in laboratories where they are accessible for genetic engineering, and this engineering can exert some control over human evolution.
2. *In vitro* fertilization clinics in a number of countries are freezing human embryos.
3. A pioneer in *in vitro* fertilization has announced plans to work on the division of human embryos.
4. Commmercial firms in the United States are offering the rental of surrogate mothers (breeders) to paying customers, some of whom are infertile couples, others, single men.
5. Physicians have artificially inseminated women, flushed embryos out of them and transferred those embryos to other women, and a commercial firm plans to set up a network of clinics around the United States offering this "service."
6. Sex predetermination clinics are providing services to couples who want boy babies.

The Reproduction Revolution we are in the midst of brings to us and to all future generations changes more profound than those brought by the Industrial Revolution. We need, each of us, to reflect on these technologies and, as a Brazilian friend of mine wrote to me, not accept them as if they were merely another brand of Coca-Cola™ in the supermarket.

Reflections on the reality of the new technologies, of course, will not be enough. O.K., we can *consider* reality. We can discuss it. That is fair. But we need more than reality. We need truth. And to arrive at truth, we will have to look at what interests me most: Women's experience. Women's perceptions. Unreality. What the king can not see.

NOTES

1. Among those common motives for wanting children are a desire to relive their own childhoods, to become parents as a "rite of passage" to adulthood, and to have children in one's life for sheer love of children.

2. A tiny sample of that literature: Scully, Diane. 1980. *Men Who Control Women's Health*. Boston: Houghton Mifflin Co.; Spender, Dale. 1982. *Women of Ideas*. London: Routledge and Keagan Paul. Spender, 1980; Corea, 1985a; Daly, Mary. 1968. *The Church and Second Sex*. New York: Harper Colophon Books; Daly, Mary. 1978. *Gyn/Ecology*. Boston: Beacon Press: Dworkin, Andrea. 1976. *Our Blood*. New York: Perigee; Dworkin, 1981; Ruth, Sheila. 1980. *Issues in Feminism: A First Course in Women's Studies*. 1980. Boston: Houghton Mifflin Co.; Morgan, Robin. 1984. *Sisterhood Is Global*. Garden City, New York: Anchor Books.

3. David Smith, a gynecologist in an IVF program at London's Royal Free Hospital, has acknowledged that the uterus may be traumatized during the embryo transfer. See: *Medical World News*, "Test tube baby efforts reviewed in Britain," Nov. 24, 1980. p. 49.

REFERENCES

Bruce, Judith and S. Bruce Schearer. 1983, Feb. *Contraceptives and developing countries: the role of barrier methods*. International Symposium on Research on the Regulation of Human Fertility. Stockholm, Sweden.

Burton, Barbara A. 1985, March. "Contentious issues of infertility therapy: A Consumer View." Paper presented before the Australian Family Planning Conference.

Corea, Gena. 1985a. *The Hidden Malpractice*. New York: Harper & Row.

———. 1985b. *The Mother Machine*. New York: Harper & Row.

——— and Susan Ince. 1985, July 3. "IVF a game for losers at half of U.S. clinics." *Medical Tribune*.

Dworkin, Andrea. 1981. *Pornography: Men Possessing Women*. New York: Perigee.

Frye, Marilyn. 1983. *The Politics of Reality: Essays in Feminist Theory*. Trumansburg, New York: The Crossing Press.

Graebner, William. 1984, August. "Doing the world's unhealthy work: the fiction of free choice." *The Hastings Center Report*. 28-37.

Hanmer, Jalna. 1985. "Transforming consciousness: women and the new reproductive technologies." *Man-Made Women*. London: Hutchinson.

Hartmann, Betsy. 1987. *Reproductive Rights and Wrongs: The Global Politics of Population Control and Contraceptive Choice*. New York: Harper and Row.

Keye, William R. 1982, March. "Strategy for avoiding iatrogenic infertility." *Contemporary Ob/Gyn* 19:185-195.

Muasher, Suheil J. and Jairo E. Garcia and Howard W. Jones, Jr. 1984. "Experience with diethylstilbestrol-exposed infertile women in a program of in vitro fertilization." *Fertility and Sterility* 42(1):20-24.

Murdoch, Anna. 1985, April 10. "When IVF is a lost labor." *The Age*. (Australia) 18.

OGN, 1980, June 1. "PID epidemic today, infertility tomorrow." *Ob Gyn News*.

Oppenheimer, W. 1959. "Prevention of pregnancy by the Grafenberg ring method: a re-evaluation after 28 years experience." *American Journal of Obstetrics and Gynecology* 87:446-454.

Richart, Ralph M. 1981, Jan. "Ovarian Abscesses in IUD Wearers." *Contemporary Ob/Gyn*.

Rothman, Barbara Katz. 1985. *The Tentative Pregnancy*. New York: Viking Press.

Spender, Dale. 1980. *Man-Made Language*. London: Routledge and Kegan Paul Ltd.

Stamm, Walter E. and Susan Kaetz and King K. Holmes. 1982. "Clinical training in venereology in the United States and Canada." *Journal of the American Medical Association* 248(16):2020-2024.

Wiesner, Paul J. 1979, April 27. "Dear Colleague" letter. Washington, D.C. U.S. Printing Office 1979-642-979/6346. Available for $2 from the Boston Women's Health Book Collective, 47 Nichols Avenue, Watertown, MA 02172.

Women in Medicine. 1984. Unpublished and untitled submission to the Warnock Commission. London.

Reproductive Technology and the Commodification of Life

Barbara Katz Rothman

SUMMARY. This paper suggests that the key unifying concept in the development and application of new reproduction technology has been the increasing commodification of life — treating people and parts of people as marketable commodities. This commodification process is made most dramatically clear in (1) prenatal diagnosis, in which the fetus is treated as a product subject to quality control measures and women are treated as producers without emotional tie to their products and (2) in so-called "surrogacy" arrangements in which an actual price tag is placed on pregnancy, and women sell both their "labor" and their "product."

The issues that confront us in reproduction these days are indeed complex. They involve new technology, old technology and no technology at all. We confront the newer questions raised by prenatal diagnosis and selective abortion, by *in vitro* fertilization, by something we are calling "surrogate" motherhood, and we face the older questions raised by adoption. It is a bewildering, frightening, challenging array.

Is there any way of organizing our thoughts about these issues, of seeing connections between the disparate techniques and questions? I believe that medicine has, this time unwittingly, supplied us with a key to all of this. The key is not another technology, but a phrase, a bit of language, words that open up and lay bare the underlying

The author wishes to thank Rosalyn Weinman Schram for her insight and wording on this issue.

95

ideology which unites our reproductive technology. The phrase is "the products of conception." It is medical language for what you get when sperm joins egg — in a loving waiting mother, in a frightened teenager, in a hired woman, or in a petrie dish — the results are "the products of conception."

Interesting phrase, that. It is really a fine term for what we're talking about. Because in fact we are talking about products and a production process. We are facing the expansion of an ideology that treats people as objects, as commodities. It is an ideology that enables us to see not motherhood, not parenthood, but the creation of a commodity, a baby. We are involved now in the fixing of price tags to the separate parts of the reproductive process. We are negotiating the prices for bodily parts, bodily fluids, human services, energy and lives, as we produce "valuable" babies, "precious" babies.

This is the theme that I see running through all of the issues in the new, and in the old, reproductive technology. Sometimes the theme comes right up to the surface, and we hear and read actual dollar figures: so many thousands of dollars for each *in vitro* attempt, $10,000 as the current market rate for a "surrogate" mother-for-hire, $20,000 to adopt a baby from one country, $15,000 from another. Sometimes the language of commodification, of pricing, goes back under again, and we talk vaguely about the "costs" and the "burdens" of rearing people with disabilities, how much we are "spared" with selective abortion. The talk of money and dollars comes to the fore and recedes to the background, but always, through it all, when we talk about reproduction these days we are talking about the commodification of life. It is not altogether surprising in this society at this time, that this is indeed the approach we take to reproduction: some would claim that this is the approach we take to virtually everything in the United States. We talk about costs and prices, bottom lines and net gains, what things are worth.

This commodification process is very clearly seen in the notion of "surrogate" motherhood. There we talk openly about buying services and renting body parts — as if body parts were rented without the people who surround the part, as if you could rent a woman's uterus without renting the woman. We ignore our knowledge that women are pregnant with our whole bodies, from the changes in our hair to our swollen feet, with all of our bodies and perhaps with our souls as well. We make it "simple," we make it "straightforward" and we make little jokes about "wombs for rent."

But the commodification process is not uniquely seen in surrogacy arrangements: it was there long ago when we first began to experience some "shortage" of babies for adoption. While babies are not for sale in the United States, at least not openly, we all know perfectly well that the availability of a baby for adoption has a lot to do with the amount of money in the hands of the potential adopters. And we know that adoptable babies are themselves sorted as commodities: the whiter, younger and healthier carry the highest price tags; others—the wrong color, damaged, too long on the shelf, the "seconds" of the production process—go cheaply, go begging.

And now we see the commodification process enter all pregnancies, as society encourages the development of prenatal diagnostic technology. This process, the genetic counseling, the screening and testing of fetuses, serves the function of "quality control" on the assembly line of the products of conception, separating out those products we wish to develop from those we wish to discontinue. And we see the commodification process not only in technological developments but in legal developments as well. The "wrongful life" suits, the suits claiming that a particular fetus should never have been conceived, or never brought to term, are a form of "product liability" litigation.[1] Once we see the products of conception as just that, as products, we begin to treat them as we do any other product, subject to similar scrutiny and standards.

One concern raised by the use of this developing ideology is what it does to the "products of conception" to be dealt with in this way. And so, we worry about the effects of artificial insemination with the use of sperm from paid donors, or "surrogate" motherhood and other purchasing agreements, on the children thus created. Certainly, some worry about the fetus and its "right to life," with or without disabilities. But my chief concern lies elsewhere: I want us to think about what this commodification process does to all of us, to us as a society, to us as individuals, and most particularly what it does to women as mothers.

Let me take as an illustration of my concern what has happened in another area of life with the process of commodification. It is not only reproduction that has been commodified, not only eggs and sperm that we sell. Consider what we have done with blood. In the United States we buy and sell blood. In Richard Titmuss' fine book THE GIFT RELATIONSHIP (1972), the author explores the consequences of the commodification of blood, of turning blood into a purchasable product, and compares American and British blood banking systems. In the United States blood needs to be purchased. One gives blood either for cash, in the most straightforward, crass example of commodification, or in the slightly round-about way of donating blood for blood insurance. In England, by contrast, blood is freely available: one is not charged for its use and not paid for its donation. Thus the giving of blood is a purely altruistic act. The payment of blood-money removes from us as blood donors the right to be altruistic, the right to give freely.

The argument that Titmuss makes does not draw upon the "rights of blood," does not concern itself with the moral value of the blood per se, but rather with the moral value of the giving and selling — what it does to *us*, not to the blood, to commodify blood.

When we look at slides of the products of conception, when the new technology shows us what those newly formed pre-embryo cells look like, we see cells: one, two, four, eight cell clusters, looking as if they lie on a bed of sand before us in their magnified banality. To the non-scientists among us, we might just as well be looking at blood cells, at plant cells, at anything and at nothing. Let us look not at the cells, and not even at the people those cells might become, but rather let us look at the society that prices those cells, and most especially at the women in whose bodies those cells must grow.

I will conclude by briefly considering two of the groups of women most directly affected by the commodification process in reproduction: first, the mothers awaiting prenatal diagnostic testing; and secondly, the women hired as "surrogates."

What happens to women who are undergoing the quality control process of prenatal diagnosis, women who do not yet know if they are mothers, or if they are carriers of something we are going to call a defective fetus and ask them to abort? In my interviews with women caught in this process (Rothman 1986), I saw the development of the "tentative pregnancy," the condition in which a woman acknowledges her wanted pregnancy, accepts the roles and rituals of pregnancy, but knows she may not be having the baby she wants, but the abortion she dreads. I have seen how these women suffer, how they recoil from the movement of fetuses slated for abortion, begging of their bellies, "Baby please, please don't move." I have seen how they cannot maintain the medical language, the needed distancing, but feel the baby within as a baby, as their baby, and when they know they have to end the pregnancy — for good and strong reasons — they use not the language of abortion and termination, but the language of infanticide, of murder and killing, of grief and responsibility. Motherhood resists commodification.

And what does it do to women who "rent" their wombs, to the women we ask to carry within them a baby they are to believe is not theirs? Some women seem to adapt well to the situation: they stand there large with child and say, "This is not my baby. This is someone else's baby. I will birth it and give it up without a qualm." These women have accepted the alienation of the worker from the product of her labor: the baby like any other commodity does not belong to the producer but to the purchaser. But some women do not adapt so well. Some women, like Mary Beth Whitehead, say they agreed to sell an egg, to rent a womb, but in the course of pregnancy and birth realize that that was not what was required. What was required was that they sell a child, sell their baby. That they cannot do. Those are the women who refuse to be workers, who find that they cannot commodify their motherhood, cannot fix price tags on their babies. As Whitehead said, "I looked at $10,000 and I looked at my daughter, and there's no question. This child is my child just like my other children."

So what are we doing to ourselves as we commodify reproduction, create it in the image of all production, aim for "state of the art" babies? We put a price tag on our lives and our love, learn, as they say, "the price of everything and the value of nothing."

Here we are, actively pricing motherhood — it costs about $1,000 to purchase a spare embryo, another $10,000 to "rent a womb," and there we have it. What is the meaning, what the value of motherhood? $11,000 on the open market. And once the priceless is priced, market considerations take over. How long before the brokers in this business, the men who have books of women's pictures to show prospective purchasers, follow the cattle industry in seeking higher profits? With cattle, profits have been increased by planting more valuable embryos in less valuable breeders. Can we look forward to baby farms, with white embryos grown in young and poor Third-World mothers? Price goes down, labor costs are saved, and profit goes up.

But who profits here? In whose interests are we developing our technology? Where is the profit in commodifying life?

REFERENCES

Titmuss, R. 1972. *The Gift Relationship: From Human Blood to Social Policy.* New York: Vintage.
Rothman, B. K. 1986. *The Tentative Pregnancy: Prenatal Diagnosis and the Future of Motherhood.* New York. Viking/Penguin.

Moral Pioneers:
Women, Men and Fetuses on a
Frontier of Reproductive Technology

Rayna Rapp

SUMMARY. As one of the new reproductive technologies, amniocentesis is rapidly becoming routinized, especially for pregnant
women in their mid-thirties and older. Prenatal diagnosis has been
evaluated medically, economically, and bioethically. But we know
very little about how pregnant women and their families who use, or
might use, this new technology respond to its benefits and burdens.
This article reports on a two-year field study in New York City.
Responses of genetic counselors, a multicultural patient population
using and refusing amniocentesis, women who had received "positive" diagnoses, and families with children who have the conditions
that can now be diagnosed prenatally were all elicited through par-
ticipant-observation. My goal in this study is to assess the social
impact and cultural meaning of one new reproductive technology.

Each year, scores of thousands of American women choose to
monitor their pregnancies for prenatal disabilities via amniocentesis, and the number is rapidly growing. Indeed, the exact number of
amniocenteses performed each year is unknown: in the same year
(1983) three different government sources suggested 40,000,

The field work on which this essay is based was funded by the National Science
Foundation and the National Endowment for the Humanities. I am grateful to
both. I also want to thank the many women and their families who took this
inquiry to heart, sharing their amniocentesis stories with me. The health professionals who aided my work have all believed in the importance of understanding
their patients' experiences. I'm grateful for their trust. Many audiences of feminists—scholars and activists—have sharpened my work through the questions
they have posed. Without them, the context for this inquiry would be immeasur-
ably impoverished.

101

80,000, and 120,000. The lack of a "ballpark estimate" should alert us to the fact that we are observing a medical technology which is becoming widespread under conditions of a "free market economy," without much centralized monitoring. In 1950, there were only a handful of genetic centers in the USA; now, there are over 500 where amniocentesis is performed. And while the technology was initially developed to monitor Down Syndrome (a leading cause of mental retardation, worldwide), it can now detect about 200 inherited conditions, most of them quite rare recessive diseases. Unless otherwise indicated by family health history, a standard amniocentesis is performed to look for chromosome defects and open neural tube defects, and not for more arcane conditions.

Those recommended for the test include women whose families already have a member with a condition that can now be detected prenatally; people from ethnically specific populations in which the risk of certain recessively transmitted genetic diseases is elevated (Tay-Sachs among people of Azkenazi Jewish descent; sickle cell anemia among those of African descent, for example); and "older" pregnant women. "Older" is, however, a social, and not a simply biological construct: while the incidence of Down Syndrome live-born babies goes steadily up throughout a woman's childbearing years, the cut-off age for the test has varied considerably. As amniocentesis becomes safer, the age at which it is offered has dropped from 40 to 38 to 35, and it is now hovering in the lower thirties. There is no automatically "correct" age at which the test is indicated: the current suggestion that women 35 years of age and older have the test while pregnant springs not from any jump in the incidence of Down Syndrome, but from the intersection of two epidemiological statistics: at 35, the incidence of liveborn babies with Down Syndrome is about one in 360; amniocentesis is considered a very safe test, but it does add an additional risk of miscarriage to the pregnancies of women who undergo the procedure. That added risk is one-third of one percent, or one in 330, a number which approximates the risk of bearing a liveborn child with Down Syndrome for 35-year old women. If the technology caused one less miscarriage per thousand, the age at which it is recommended would drop considerably. And as new technologies like the chorionic villus sampling technique, and eventually, maternal/fetal blood centrifuges become clinically available, the population recommended to use prenatal diagnosis is likely to expand.[1] We are thus witnessing the intersection of a routinizing technology with an epidemiological pattern, and not just a biologically absolute threshold of pregnancy risk.

Amniocentesis and its related technologies (like diagnostic ultrasound) are part of the new reproductive technologies—*in vitro* and *in vivo* fertilization, embryo transfer, embryo replacement, donor insemination—which have been much touted in the popular press as "playing god" with baby-making. Are we replacing mothers with machines? fathers with doctors? nature by mechanical culture? How are these technologies changing the experiences of pregnancy, of becoming a parent, and of family life?

In studying amniocentesis as an anthropologist, I hope to restore a social context, and probe the cultural meaning, of one new reproductive technology as it is becoming routinized. Moreover, I am examining one aspect of biological science in American culture, and of medicine as the applied arena in which most Americans routinely experience scientific language and technology. Genetics holds a privileged position in this medical discourse, for it has fired the popular as well as the scientific imagination in ways that are deeply consonant with some of our most cherished beliefs in American culture. In thinking about the historical discourse on biometry, Mendelianism, eugenics, sociobiology and, now, the new genetic engineering technologies, we see that genetics provides metaphors of human perfectability, and definitions of the individual as holding within itself its own potentialities. Medical attention to the individual reflects deeply-held cultural beliefs. While legal and medical expert definitions of personhood increasingly prevail, they are based on notions of individuality which fit well with the historical roots of American culture.

The problems of prenatal diagnosis have been discussed by geneticists (who assess the potentials and limits of their technologies); by health economists (who use cost-benefit analysis to tell us that it is cheaper to screen scores of thousands of pregnancies than to support the services required for each liveborn baby with a genetic disability) and by bioethicists (who have raised important questions concerning informed consent, the eugenic potentials of amniocentesis, and parents' rights to know and not know). But what is stunning when one enters the discourse on prenatal diagnosis as an anthropologist (and, in my case, I was then a pregnant woman) is that all the audible voices belong to experts. And the experts are predominantly male and white. Silent are the multicultural voices of the women and their families who use, or might use, the new technology. We have very little sense of what their experiences, choices, responses, and images of amniocentesis are all about. And what little research exists concerning users of amniocentesis is constrained by the assumptions of methodological individualism: the personalities of pregnant women have been assessed for anxiety and information retention, and how rationally they respond to risk factors. But no one has tried to situate their experiences in a larger social picture. Yet when we step back, it is apparent that reproductive "choices" are far more than individual, or psychological. Broad demographic, sexual, reproductive (and non-reproductive) patterns are ultimately *social* patterns, contextualized by the rationalities of class, race, ethnicity, sex, religious background, family and reproductive history, and not simply by individual "risks and benefits." It is this larger context I seek to identify and interpret in my fieldwork as an anthropologist.

While nationally, amniocentesis is becoming a ritual of pregnancy mainly for highly educated, urbanized sectors of the white middle classes, the situation in New York City is somewhat different. I am presently conducting field work through the Prenatal Diagnosis Laboratory (PDL) of the City of New York, which was set up explicitly to offer amniocentesis to low-income (and thus, disproportionally Afro-American and Hispanic) women beginning in 1978. The lab accepts medicaid and has a sliding scale fee which begins at no-cost. It works through 24 City hospitals (both voluntary and municipal), and it initially made counseling available in several languages. The samples of amniotic fluid it collects come from women whose ethnic backgrounds are approximately one-third Afro-American, one-third Hispanic, and one-third white. About half are clinic (low-income), about half are private patients. From an anthropological perspective, it is thus a "social laboratory" as well as a biological one.

My fieldwork focuses on seven contexts and constituencies. In exploring multiple perspectives on the meaning of prenatal diagnosis, I hope to construct a social and political understanding of one new reproductive technology. One of my salient goals is to demedicalize the discourse on amniocentesis, helping to make its implications available for discussion by the people who use, or might use it. While this complex story must await a longer presentation, in this article I shall name the contexts in which my research occurs, indicating some of the social and cultural issues that each reveals.

IN THE LABORATORY

With the support of PDL's Chief Geneticist, I was a participant-observer at the Lab for two months, watching geneticists, genetic counselors, lab technicians and support staff work in dense and daily interaction. In addition to conducting extensive interviews with both professional and support staff, I followed apprentice technicians through their training, so as to understand both the language and labor of genetics. Using an "ethnography of science" perspective, I observed the practices of ordinary science: scientific personnel making meaning, rehearsing rituals, negotiating significance, as well as "producing results" (Latour & Woolgar 1979; Knorr-Cetina & Mulkay 1982; Goodfield 1981).

Given the powerful place science in general, and genetics in particular, currently hold in late 20th century American culture, I focus on the metaphors used in the translation of one cutting edge of research into clinical practice and public policy. Those metaphors are, of course, quite gender-laden in their descriptions of hierarchy and reciprocity within DNA and chromosomes, and throughout medicine itself (Hubbard 1982; Minden 1984).

At the sociological level, the labors involved in prenatal diagnosis are women's work. Not only are pregnant women the clients for this new reproductive service, but virtually all the workers in this "industry" are female, as well. Medical geneticists working in this field are disproportionately women. While men predominate on the research frontier of genetic engineering, women find medical genetics to be more hospitable. It provides 9-to-5 working hours without late-night emergencies and is thus compatible with the domestic sexual division of labor. More than 98% of all genetic counselors are female. While they are experts in a technical and rapidly-changing science, counselors are situated in the medical hierarchy like social workers, and paid as such. Most lab technicians are women, as well. This work is often cited as appropriately "feminine" because it focuses on pregnancy, and does not disrupt family responsibilities. A new field of employment at the cutting edge of genetics thus emerges with job descriptions, prestige and pay scales that reproduce familiar gender hierarchies.

In the laboratory, genetic technicians peer through microscopes, constructing karyotypes, searching for atypical chromosomal patterns. They do so constrained by a work structure which separates fetal cells from babies, blood samples from pregnant women, diagnoses from family trauma. It is important to examine both the benefits and the boundaries of the scientific division of labor as it constructs amniocentesis.

GENETIC COUNSELORS

Genetic counseling is a profession in formation (Rollnick 1984; Reed 1974; Kevles 1985). In its scant fifteen-year history, the field has trained a new group of predominantly white, middle-class female health professionals to explain chromosomes and genetic disability to lay audiences. The initial wave of genetic counselors tended to be well-educated suburban housewives raising their children first, and then returning to the job market. Many lived near Sarah Lawrence College, in Westchester County, New York where the first training program opened its doors in 1971. Recently, a second wave of genetic counselors has begun to appear on the job market. Younger, a bit more ethnically and linguistically diverse, second wave counselors tend to have postponed childbearing in favor of careers. These background factors are important, as both waves of counselors are unlikely to have experienced the technology they now offer to other women. And their own experiences surrounding female work and family life necessarily inform their attitudes toward pregnant patients.

I have conducted interviews with thirty genetic counselors, at least one from every health facility in New York City where amniocentesis is offered. I have also worked closely with the PDL counseling team during a two-year period, observing their intake interviews at hospitals throughout New York City. Genetic counselors are quick to identify the ethical complexity of providing prenatal information and health services, including abortion services, to women of diverse ethnic, racial, linguistic and religious backgrounds. They are trained to be empathic as they convey statistics, and to practice Rogerian therapy, a non-interventionist technique aimed at helping the patient to make up her own mind. Yet genetic counselors all know how perilous the position of value-free counseling is. On the one hand, they are always making linguistic code-switches as they determine what sort and how much information a pregnant woman needs and can use. On the other, all the information that woman receives comes directly from the counselor, as she is unlikely to have a "folk model" of most of the diseases and risks associated with amniocentesis. Not so with other aspects of pregnancy, which are also discussed informally, amongst kin, neighbors, and friends, in a popular, as well as a medical voice.

So the genetic counselor really is the gate keeper between science and social experience, regulating the quantity and quality of the information on which decisions will be made. In their work, genetic counselors identify with and serve pregnant women, while representing the universal claims of science. At stake in their profession is the technological transformation of pregnancy and maternal "choice."

DURING COUNSELING

For two years, I have observed hundreds of intake interviews in three City hospitals where genetic counselors explain inheritance patterns and amniocentesis to a polyglot, multicultural patient population. Here, genetic counselors elicit a great deal of information from their patients — ethnic background (to know if they are at risk for any ethnically specific disease, like Thalassemia, Tay-Sachs, or sickle-cell anemia), occupation (to check for hazardous exposures), method of payment, as well as personal, reproductive, and family health histories. I observe code switching ("baby" versus "fetus"; "tummy" versus "womb" or "uterus"; "waters" versus "amniotic fluid") as counselors deal in dizzying succession with Guccibriefcased husband-wife-law-teams, Dominican high school drop outs, and Seventh Day Adventists from Harlem. I observe not only what questions are asked, but what questions are unasked, as well. Thus, a middle-class, professional couple queries whether the husband's Aunt Hannah, who had a perfectly healthy baby at 45, is included in the counselor's health statistics. But a clinic patient waiting three hours to keep her appointment may respond to the query, "Do you have any questions to ask me?" with, "Where's the Medicaid office?" And a pregnant black teenager with sickle trait may confront the counselor with a folk explanation: as the last child, she has a touch of trait because all last children do. Or a recently-migrated Haitian couple may reject amniocentesis because they've never heard of Down Syndrome, or "mongolism," for which no word appears to exist in their native Creole.[2]

In a 45-minute session, conversations (and silences) are rich with possible communication, and miscommunication. Here, the local meaning of a pregnancy, a fetus, heredity, and technology are all under negotiation. And the language of science often confronts polyglot dialects of daily life.

AT HOME

The waiting period between amniocentesis and its results is a very long and stressful one. The test can't be administered before the 16th week of pregnancy, when enough fluid has accumulated for a successful and safe tap. The lab work includes a lengthy cell-growth period, and tedious karyotyping, which take three to four weeks. And results must be known before the 24th week of pregnancy, the legal limit in the State of New York for termination of a pregnancy, should a woman discover she is bearing a disabled fetus and want to abort. During this stressful waiting period, women and their families are often quite willing to speak with friendly outsiders about their experiences with amniocentesis.

In visiting at home with a selected sample of forty-five Afro-American, Hispanic, and white families (stratified by occupation and payment method to get a class-diverse picture), I have queried how women feel about the test, the health care professionals, and the information they are given. My data includes people's responses to knowing, or not knowing, the sex of the fetus.[3] I also probe for images of pregnancy, disability, and dependency. Most people, for example, can articulate a description of Down Syndrome. But fewer know about spina bifida (neural tube defects) for which the test is also done, and almost none know about other chromosome problems.

Pregnant women in ethnically-specific populations confront not only the diseases but the health politics, of the conditions for which they may be at risk in deciding to use amniocentesis. Tay-Sachs disease, for example, is most prevalent among Jews of Azkenazi descent, and sickle cell anemia is most prevalent among people of African descent. The health consequences of the diseases vary enormously. The first is inevitably fatal for children; the second produces a condition which can vary from extremely mild to painful and life-threatening. And the history of screening programs and community education varies radically for the two diseases. Responses to being offered a prenatal screen, and subsequent abortion of an affected fetus are quite different. While Jews of Azkenazi descent are likely to go for screening, and to abort all affected fetuses, there is much less compliance with the test in Black communities, and abortion rates following sickling detection are probably about 40%.

Above all, home interviews reveal how women think about pregnancy with the advent of this technology. My data centers on the connections, responsibilities and maternal identities pregnant women express in the context of their social, rather than their medical, biographies. Attitudes about abortion and sick children are central to this section of my work.

Does amniocentesis offer women a "window of control," or an anxiety-provoking responsibility, or both? Is there a transition for those who use prenatal diagnosis between an image of mothers as all-nurturant, self-sacrificing madonnas, and mothers as agents of quality control on the reproductive production line? Neither is a simple image, for both are constructed by interests with which women may come into conflict. But the second reveals the limits of selflessness that mothers are alleged to have. It is perhaps part of a larger transformation of the meaning of motherhood in an age of high female labor-force participation rates; later marriages; high divorce rates; smaller families and later childbearing (at least for some Americans), and an increased use of legal abortion. In this context, a decision to bear or not to bear a child with serious health problems in a society which provides meager services for disabled children and their families takes on new meanings.

POSITIVE DIAGNOSIS

While 98% of the women who undergo amniocentesis will receive the good news that their fetuses are free of the conditions for which they have been tested, 2% will face the distressing news of fetal disability. Medical discourse here systematically inverts maternal experience: "positive" diagnoses have enormously negative impacts on the lives of women who receive them. Yet we know very little about the benefits and burdens of the information this reproductive technology reveals from the perspective of the women who use it (Blumberg et al. 1975; Jones et al. 1984; Furlong & Black 1984). Twenty-nine retrospective interviews focus on the moral and cultural reasoning of women who with their support networks had to make a decision to continue or end a pregnancy science had revealed to be affected.

While most women receiving positive diagnoses go on to abort, the solutions people chose are in part dependent on the specific diagnosis and their cultural background. Down Syndrome, for example, carries an abortion rate of close to 100%, but the sex-chromosome anomalies are aborted at rates that are probably between 50 and 75%. And sickle-cell anemia is cause for abortion in about 40% of the women who receive it as a fetal diagnosis. Interviews with women and their families who had to make a difficult decision to continue or end a pregnancy that technology revealed to be affected point to the cultural diversity of both problems and solutions. Similar decisions may illuminate very different cultural premises. For example, two couples who aborted after receiving a prenatal diagnosis of Klinefelter's Syndrome (XXY, a sex chromosome anomaly) gave these differing rationales: one said, "If he was gonna be slow, if he wasn't gonna have a shot at being President, that's not the baby we wanted." The other said, "With all the problems a child has to face, it isn't fair to add this burden." The first couple was middle-class and professional; the second, recent migrants and very poor.

Prior knowledge, medical networks, and support systems also enter into the decision to end or continue an affected pregnancy. And religious background is clearly significant here. Virtually all the Jews in my sample described technology in general, and amniocentesis in particular, as a humane addition to their lives, despite the pain of ending a desired pregnancy. Other groups were more ambivalent. And attitudes towards abortion are connected to religious practices in complex, mediated ways. Many Hispanic women, for example, report multiple early abortions, but consider *late* abortion to be a sin. Here, a finely-honed set of female-centered distinctions is being developed as popular theology. The local meanings of pregnancy, maternity, parental love, and adult gender identity shape the decisions surrounding abortion or the birth of a disabled child.

Despite their diversity, retrospective interviews also reveal the common depths of isolation inherent in pursuing the consequences of this new reproductive technology. No one interviewed had ever met another woman who sustained this same experience of "positive" diagnosis. This is not true for other reproductive losses like abortion, miscarriage, stillbirth, all of which have social as well as medical aspects that can be located. Technology here creates a traumatic experience which is so deeply medicalized and privatized that its social shape has yet to be excavated, and a cultural language for its description is yet to be found.

PARADOXES OF DISABILITY

Some of the same conditions that can now be screened prenatally can also be better managed postnatally due to both medical and social advances. Paradoxically, children with Down Syndrome and spina bifida have much better survival rates, and can lead much richer lives, than was possible twenty years ago. Down Syndrome, for example, no longer leads to institutionalization. Most DS children now receive infant stimulation, and are able to function as only mildly to moderately retarded. Many go to school, learning to read and write. Children with spina bifida frequently didn't survive unless their condition was extremely mild ("passing" as normal), but now, infant surgery and physical therapy have helped to create a generation of young adults who have grown up with this condition. We have yet to hear their voices very directly, but surely, some are represented in the disability rights movement (Saxton 1984 and in this volume; Asch 1986; Asch & Fine 1984).

In order to understand the social, rather than the medical, implications of giving birth to a child with a genetic disability, I have spent almost three years as a participant-observer in a support group for parents of children with Down Syndrome. From scores of parent-activists, I have learned about the "courtesy stigmas" involved in having a disabled child (Goffman 1963; Darling 1979; Featherstone 1980). Support group members are disproportionately white and upper-middle class. Consequently, I have also interviewed fifteen Afro-American and Hispanic parents of genetically disabled children, located through an infant stimulation program.

Families whose children have the same conditions that amniocentesis now diagnoses prenatally speak counterdiscourses to medical authority. Here, religion, ethnicity, class and family history powerfully shape responses to having a child with a genetically stigmatized condition. Reflections on the meaning of maternity and paternity and the value of children are embedded in the stories parents of the disabled tell as they transform medical diagnosis into the social fabric of daily life. Strategies for coping and making cultural meaning through a life crisis and family transformation vary enormously. The benefits of a self-help learning network may work best for those who are most comfortable with medical labels as part of their self-definitions. These tend to be white, middle-class families. Many parents in the Down Syndrome support group refer collectively to "our kids," for example. But a Black mother of a child with the same condition said, "My kid's got a heart problem, my kid's gonna be slow. First let me deal with that, love him for that, then I'll check out this Down Syndrome thing."

REFUSERS

About 50% of clinic patients and about 10% of private patients break their appointments for genetic counseling. Of the 1000 women counseled by the PDL genetic counselors each year, about 750 go on to amniocentesis, and 250 do not. Of those small numbers receiving a positive diagnosis, an even smaller number decides not to abort. It is important to locate and listen to those who refuse to use a technology in the process of routinization, removing themselves from the conveyor belt of its assumptions and options anywhere along the line. The reasons for refusing amniocentesis are many; religious beliefs, non-scientific constructions of pregnancy and motherhood, distrust of the medical system, fear of miscarriage. The commentary of refusers provides clues to the cultural contradictions involved in the technological transformation of pregnancy. Low-income Afro-American women, for example, often expressed a "home grown" sense of statistics which varied radically from the sensibilities of middle-class couples. When a woman has birthed four other children, comes from a family of eight, and all her sisters and neighbors have had similar histories, she has seen scores of babies born without recognizable birth defects. To contrast these experiences with a number produced by a lady in a white coat proclaiming that the risk of a baby with a birth defect is steadily rising with each pregnancy requires a leap of faith in abstract reasoning. Among middle-class professional families, however, childbearing is likely to be delayed, and the counselor is discussing a first, or at most, a second pregnancy. Children are likely to be scarce throughout the network of the professional couple. To them, one-in-three-hundred sounds like a large and present risk, while for the low-income mother of four, the same number may appear very distant and small. Moreover, chromosome defects seem a weak explanation for the problems that children may suffer. One Haitian father, firmly rejecting prenatal testing on his wife's behalf, said, "The counselor says the baby could be born retarded. They always say Haitian children are retarded. What is this retarded? Many Haitian children are said to be retarded in the public schools. If we send them to the Haitian Academy (a community-based private school) they learn just fine." In his experience, chromosomes don't loom large as an explanatory force, when compared to ongoing prejudices and labels already present in the lives of the children of his community.

Science speaks a language of universal authority. Diverse women express their gender consciousness, and the core meanings of reproduction in polyglot, multicultural voices. The analysis and interpretation of this tension illuminates one aspect of late 20th century

American culture, where science and technology make powerful claims on the transformation of pregnancy and personhood. At stake is the cultural negotiation of gender and parental practices, in a world shaped by both social diversity, and scientific hegemony. Until we locate and listen to the discourses of those women who encounter and interpret a new reproductive technology in their own lives, we cannot evaluate it beyond the medical model. Whether amniocentesis represents social control, or mitigation of female subordination, or both, is a question to which only local and unstable responses may be given. It cannot be settled by recourse to a universal explanation, as if all women held similar interests in the problems of pregnancy, or of disabled children.

The perspectives of feminist scholarship on the one hand, and the women's health movement, on the other, suggest that the lived experiences of reproduction reflect far more than medical progress and problems. When examined from these more cultural and political perspectives, we begin to see the shifting meaning of motherhood implied in our national struggles for reproductive rights, and the cultural diversity in women's ability to control the conditions under which they do and don't mother children. We badly need an analysis from the perspective of women and their families in which reproductive rights will not be pitted against disability rights. Beyond the Reagan neonatal hotlines, and the attempt to make second trimester abortion illegal in part by using disabled fetuses as icons of maternal responsibility gone awry, lies a terrain we need to explore. In it, I hope to describe a political and cultural logic by which we can and must defend both access to high quality medical care for pregnant women, including access to abortion when and if they choose it, while at the same time destigmatizing disability, and defending the special needs and services for people who cannot "get ahead" in a society where autonomy and independence are so central to the ideological definitions of personhood.

NOTES

1. Chorionic villus sampling is a first-trimester prenatal diagnostic test. A sample of pre-placental tissue containing fetal cells is removed through a trans-cervical procedure. It can be read directly, without lengthy laboratory culturing. Results are thus available by the tenth week of pregnancy. More widely used abroad, the test is still considered experimental in the United States, in part be-

cause it causes a higher rate of miscarriage than amniocentesis does. It is increasingly available under "study conditions," in major medical centers. Maternal/fetal blood centrifuges are not yet clinically available, but may become a potentially powerful diagnostic technique in the future. A useful blood centrifuge would have to discriminate between the maternal blood supply, and the small number of fetal blood cells within it. In principle, such a test could be done at the time of a first, positive pregnancy test, given the woman information about her fetus' chromosomal status at the moment she discovered she was pregnant.

2. The incidence of Down Syndrome appears to be invariant, worldwide (Hook 1981). In a country which suffers the worst health statistics in the Western hemisphere, where the infant mortality rate is close to 50%, and healthy as well as fragile babies may rapidly fall ill and die of unexplained causes, it is not surprising that the characteristic physical signs of Down's (tongue, eyes, hair, palm creases, muscle looseness, etc.) are not recognized as a "syndrome."

3. See Hanmer (1981) and Corea (1985) for important discussions of sex selection via prenatal diagnosis. Rothman (1985) has a thoughtful chapter on the implications of knowing fetal sex for parental attitudes.

4. These figures are compiled from the PDL "positive diagnosis" follow-up file.

REFERENCES

Asch, A. 1986. "Real Moral Dilemmas." *Christianity and Crisis* 46: 237-240.
Asch, A. and M. Fine. 1984. "Shared Dreams: a Left Perspective on Disability Rights and Reproductive Rights." *Radical America*.
Blumberg, B. D. et al. 1975. "Psycological Sequelae of Abortion Performed for a Genetic Indication." *American Journal of Obstetrics and Gynecology* 122:799-808.
Corea, G. 1985. *The Mother Machine*. New York: Harper and Row.
Darling, R. 1979. *Families Against Society*. Beverly Hills, CA: Sage.
Featherstone, H. 1980. *A Difference in the Family*. New York: Basic Books.
Furlong, R. and R. B. Black. 1984. "Pregnancy Termination for Genetic Indications: the Impact on Families." *Social Work in Health Care* 10:17-35.
Goffman, E. 1963. *Stigma: Notes on the Management of Spoiled Identity*. Englewood Cliffs, NJ: Prentice-Hall.
Goodfield, J. 1981. *An Imagined World*. New York: Penguin.
Hanmer, J. 1981. "Sex Predetermination, Artificial Insemination, and the Maintenance of Male-Dominated Culture" in *Women, Health and Reproduction*, edited by H. Roberts. London: Routledge and Kegan Paul.
Hook, E. B. 1981. "Rates of Chromosome Abnormalities at Different Maternal Ages." *Obstetrics and Gynecology* 58:282-285.
Hubbard, R. 1982. "The Theory and Practice of Genetic Reductionism: From Mendel's Law to Genetic Engineering" in *Towards a Liberatory Biology*, edited by S. Rose. London: Allison and Busby.
Jones, U. W. et al. 1984. "Parental Response to Mid-Trimester Therapeutic Abortion Following Amniocentesis." *Prenatal Diagnosis* 4:249-256.

Kevles, D. 1985. *In the Name of Eugenics*. New York: Knopf.
Knorr-Cetina, K. and M. Mulkay. eds. *Science Observed*. Beverly Hills, CA: Sage.
Latour, B. and S. Woolgar. 1979. *Laboratory Life*. Beverly Hills, CA: Sage.
Minden, S. 1984. "Designer Genes, a View From the Factory" in *Test-Tube Women* edited by R. Arditti, R. Duelli-Klein and S. Minden. Boston: Routledge and Kegan Paul.
Reed, S. 1974. "A Short History of Genetic Counseling." *Social Biology* 21:332-339.
Rollnick, B. 1984. "the National Society of Genetic Counselors: An Historical Perspective." *Birth Defects* 20:3-7.
Rothman, R. K. 1986. *The Tentative Pregnancy*. New York: Norton.
Saxton, M. 1984. "Born and Unborn: the Implications of Reproductive Technologies for People with Disabilities" in *Test-Tube Women* edited by R. Arditti, R. Duelli-Klein and S. Minden. Boston: Routledge and Kegan Paul.

In Vitro Fertilization
and Gender Politics

Judith Lorber

SUMMARY. From the point of view of the couple rather than the individual, infertility is in many ways a social rather than a physiological problem. Originally developed to bypass the blocked or missing Fallopian tubes of infertile women, IVF treatment has expanded to cases of male infertility due to poor sperm motility or low sperm count. In these cases, the woman may be physiologically normal reproductively, but nonetheless must undergo hormonal stimulation, sonargrams, and laparoscopy. Health care professionals so take it for granted that the most sophisticated techniques will be sought for correction of patients' problems that they rarely question patients on their motivations to undergo discomforting, expensive, and possibly dangerous treatments. Despite our culture's emphasis on motherhood, men are often the dominant partner in reproductive decisions. The increasing popularity of the use of IVF treatment in cases of male infertility is understandable in the light of men's investment in biological parenting and women's willingness to take on the physiological responsibility for treatment.

Everyday life is fearfully conservative, incomparably more conservative than technology. (Trotsky 1925)

From the point of view of the couple rather than the individual, infertility is in many ways a social rather than a physiological prob-

---

This is a revised version of a paper presented at the Feminist International Network on the New Reproductive Technologies Conference, Sweden, July, 1985, and at the Yale University Symposium, "Who Governs Reproduction?" New Haven, CT, November 1985. A shorter version was presented at the York College Conference, "Embryos, Ethics, and Eugenics: A Brave New World?" CUNY Graduate Center, November, 1985. The revision was supported by PSC-CUNY Grant 666-206.

117

lem (Calhoun and Selby 1980; Matthews and Matthews 1986; Mazor and Simons 1984; Menning 1977; Miall 1985 and 1986). One of the partners may be physically able to have a biological child with another sexual partner, but is socially precluded from doing so, at least openly. Artificial insemination by donor, adoption, or involvement with children biologically not one's own might satisfy one of the partners, but the other may feel that genetic inheritance or the pregnancy and birth experience are necessary to validate self-identity or a sense of masculinity or femininity.

The aging of the baby boom generation and the postponement of childbearing in women who want to establish careers has increased the demand for treatment of infertility in this country. The rate of infertility of this cohort may be high because they are older when they first try to conceive, and because they have had greater exposure to sexually transmitted diseases, pelvic infections, previous abortions, and occupational reproductive hazards (Aral and Cates 1983; Hatch 1984; Hull et al. 1985a).

Despite the low rates of live births recorded using IVF techniques (Corea 1985b; Jarrell et al. 1986; Seppala 1985; Soules 1985), the expansion of IVF clinics is a response to this population's sophisticated awareness of different treatments for infertility, their better education and financial status, and the pressure to exhaust every technological treatment before adoption or reconciliation to childlessness (Jones 1986; Kolata 1983; Menning 1977; Matthews and Matthews 1986; Rudkin 1977; for consumer-oriented books on the new reproductive technology, see Andrews 1984; Singer and Wells 1985; Walters and Singer 1982; Wood and Westmore 1984; also see Haug and Lavin 1983).

The demographic patterns of new reproductive technology use may reflect financial accessibility and cultural pressures more than rates of physiological infertility. Infertile couples in the United States in the past have had "a distant epidemiological profile": older, black, poorly educated, and with no biological children (Aral and Cates 1983). The couples admitted to the Yale University-New Haven Hospital IVF treatment service in 1983 were almost all white, highly educated, affluent, and 15 percent of the women and 12 percent of the men had biological children (Haseltine et al. 1985). Unlike the pattern with other new medical technologies, experimental use and routinized use of IVF have been on a population with the same demographic characteristics. Despite the high rates of infertility in poor and black populations, these groups have had a low rate of IVF use. Nonetheless, in a poll of California college students, black women had the highest proportion approving research on *in vitro* fertilization (Chico and Hartley 1981).

NEW REPRODUCTIVE TECHNIQUES

Despite its science-fiction aspects, IVF technology is not new. The first reported attempts at *in vitro* fertilization of mammalian eggs were done in Vienna in 1878, 100 years before the first baby was born from the technique (Fishel 1986). The first supposedly successful extra-corporeal conception was reported in 1934 and discussed in an editorial in the *New England Journal of Medicine* for October 21, 1937, as part of a commentary on the "brave new world." The editorial described how Pincus and Enzmann fertilized a rabbit ovum in a watch glass ". . . and reimplanting it in a doe other than the one which furnished the egg, have thus successfully inaugurated pregnancy in an unmated animal." Prophesying accurately, the editorial concluded that it would be ". . . a boon for the barren woman with closed tubes," and that with sex-typing, it will be possible ". . . to obtain a son or daughter, according to specifications, and even deliver them to women who are not their mothers" (Editorial 1937).

Human eggs were successfully fertilized *in vitro* in the late 1940s, in the United States. By 1955, the clinical potential of *in vitro* fertilization for the treatment of certain types of infertility was recognized, but the work was phased out in the United States because of the hostile social climate. Research continued with animals, and the first unequivocal mammalian birth from an extra-corporeal fertilization was reported in 1959 by Chang, an American scientist. In 1973, eggs were taken from a Mrs. Del Zio at New York Hospital, and the fluid was rushed by her husband to Columbia Presbyterian Hospital, where it was combined with his sperm and incubated. But the chief of obstetrics and gynecology at the hospital believed the process was unethical and immoral and removed the test tube from the incubator. The Del Zios sued, and

Mrs. Del Zio was awarded $50,000 for emotional stress because of the termination of the treatment. The award was paid by the chief of ob/gyn, Presbyterian Hospital, and Columbia University (Fishel 1986).

The first human test-tube baby, Louise Brown, was born on July 25, 1978, in England, and reported laconically by Steptoe and Edwards in a letter to the editor of *The Lancet* of August 12, 1978. Their clinical work was funded privately, mostly through American foundations (Edwards and Steptoe 1980). Worldwide, about 3000 babies have been born from IVF to date. The Australian register of 15 IVF programs reported major birth defects in 2.1% of 1,094 births, compared to 1.5% in the general population, a statistically significant increase (Saunders et al. 1987). However, two studies of 72 IVF children born in Australia found their psychosocial early childhood development to be normal (Mushin et al. 1986; Yovich et al. 1986).

Originally developed to bypass the blocked or missing Fallopian tubes of infertile women,[1] IVF treatment has expanded to cases of infertility due to cervical mucus hostility to sperm, long-standing infertility of unknown origin, and male infertility due to poor sperm motility or low sperm count (Cohen et al. 1984 and 1985; Cohen, Hewett and Rowland 1984; Hewett et al. 1985; Hirsch et al. 1985; Hull and Glazener 1984; Hull et al. 1984 and 1985b; Leeton et al. 1984; Lizza et al. 1984; Mahadevan 1985; Ross 1983; Sher et al. 1984; Yovich et al. 1984). In these cases, the woman may be physiologically normal reproductively, but nonetheless must undergo hormonal stimulation, sonargrams, and laparoscopy.

In a recently developed and increasingly popular protocol, gamete intra-fallopian transfer (GIFT), freshly removed oocytes are mixed with washed sperm and placed directly into a Fallopian tube without a period of incubation (Asch et al. 1984, 1985, 1986a and b). Since the GIFT procedure deposits sperm directly to the site of normal fertilization, it is seen as particularly useful in cases of severe oligospermia, cervical factor and immunologic factor infertility and ". . . an attractive alternative to IVF in cases in which the female partner of the infertile couple has at least one intact fallopian tube" (Asch et al. 1986a, p. 370). Other recent technological developments have been the use of frozen ova and embryos and the donation of ova and embryos to other infertile couples (Buster et al. 1983; Bustillo et al. 1984; Cohen et al. 1986; Edwards 1985; Freeman et al. 1986; Gorovitz 1985; Leeton and Harmon 1986; Leeton et al. 1986; Rogers and Trounson 1986; Rosenwaks 1986; Trounson 1983).

THE IVF EXPERIENCE

The fullest account of the IVF experience is the "as told to" story of "the miracle called Louise" (Brown et al. 1979). Lesley and John Brown were recommended to Steptoe by their National Health Service physician. Steptoe took them as private patients; the treatment was paid for by winnings from a football pool. John Brown's rationale for trying the experimental technique is typical of infertile couples where one partner has had a biological child with another person. He said:

> When people asked, I tried to make out it wasn't so bad for me, having had a family in my first marriage and Sharon being my child. But that wasn't how I really felt. I wanted a family just as much as Les. She was my wife, and I wanted her to have my baby. It would have made all the difference in the world to have our own child. (95)

Lesley Brown's experience will never happen again. She was not only the first successful IVF patient, but she didn't know how much of an experiment she was involved in. She said:

> I don't remember Mr. Steptoe saying his method of producing babies had ever worked, and I certainly didn't ask. I just imagined that hundreds of children had already been born through being conceived outside their mothers' wombs. . . . It just didn't occur to me that it would almost be a miracle if it worked with me. I wouldn't have believed it if Mr. Steptoe had told me straight out that, after years of trying, no one had ever had a baby from an implant. (106)

An account of those "years of trying" by the men involved describes the social situation of the early years of IVF treatment, in which every success brought media stardom (Edwards and Steptoe 1980; also cf. Fox 1959).

Reported research since then has focused on psychological profiles and reactions, usually just of the women patients (Alder 1985; Bainbridge 1982; Crowe 1985; Daniels 1986; Freeman 1985; Given et al. 1985; Greenfeld et al. 1987; Hasetltine et al. 1985; Johnston et al. 1985; Kemeter et al. 1985 and 1986; Mahlstedt and Macduff 1985; Mazure et al. 1985; Mikesell and Falk 1985; Shrednick 1983). Most of the patients are articulate, well-informed, and knowledgeable enough about the IVF process to know that the success rates are low and that when hormone levels drop, a pregnancy will not occur. The most stressful IVF trial is the first one and the one that is expected to be the last one. Emotionally, patients tend to experience a "roller coaster effect": first, the ovulation stimulation has to work; second, the retrieved eggs have to be "good" or fertilizable; third, at least one of the eggs has to be fertilized; fourth, the gamete has to mature properly; fifth, the implantation has to "take"; sixth, the hormone levels have to stay high; seventh, the pregnancy has to go to term or viability of the fetus(es); and eighth, the infants have to be normal. The part of the process least likely to succeed is the implantation. Since the best success rate occurs with two or three embryos, IVF clients have to be prepared for twins, triplets, and sometimes quadruplets.

The husband often experiences stress around the need to produce semen by masturbation under time pressure, and often in less than private circumstances. Some programs arrange for the wife to participate, and others have an on-site training program to relieve anxiety (Edwards and Purdy 1982:199). Implantation of the fertilized embryo, because it does not need anesthesia or operating rooms, is sometimes romanticized. At the Bourn Hall clinic, Steptoe and Edwards were convinced that the first IVF success was partly due to a midnight implantation. Their belief in natural biological rhythms (they did not use artificial stimulation of ovulation at the beginning) led to the ritual of night implantation, with the husband present and the wife dressing up for the occasion (Andrews 1984:133).

Other ways of relieving the stress of the two-to-three-week long protocol are to assign a social worker or nurse to give psychological support (Greenfeld et al. 1985; Harris 1986), educational talks and counseling (Appleton 1986), to encourage couples undergoing IVF treatment at the same time to form a support group (Leeton et al. 1982; Shrednick 1985), and even to donate fertilized embryos to each other (Leeton and Harmon 1986; Leeton et al. 1986; Rosenwaks, 1986; Trounson 1983).

IVF: TREATMENT OF CHOICE?

Health care professionals so take it for granted that the most sophisticated techniques will be sought for correction of patients' problems that they rarely question patients on their motivations to undergo discomforting, expensive, and possibly dangerous treatments (Hubbard 1981). Indeed, the medical perspective so imbues interactions between patients and health professionals that patients' "lifeworld" concerns and hesitations are frequently ignored or discounted (Mishler 1984; Rothman 1984; Waitzkin 1983:137-183). Infertility is routinely considered a physiological problem of the couple, even though one of the pair usually has a normally functioning reproductive system (Greil et al. 1988; Miall 1985 and 1986). Both medically and culturally, a "family" consists of a heterosexual couple with a child or children, and psychological maturity in women is supposed to include the desire to mother (Chodorow 1978; Corea 1985a; Crowe 1985; Henley 1982; Mahlstedt 1985; Mazor 1984; Menning 1982; Rossi 1977 and 1984).

A brief report of a post-treatment survey of 20 women who had been through a research-based IVF program in Edinburgh in 1984 indicated that most were positive toward the experience even though none had become pregnant (Alder 1985). A more thorough analysis of interviews of women who had IVF treatment in Australia revealed greater ambiguity toward the experience (Crowe 1985). While the women in this study wanted to become mothers, the experience of pregnancy and childbirth was not crucial. Nonetheless, "the implementation of the IVF program . . . necessitates that women perceive motherhood as a biological relationship to a child" (Crowe 1985:59). Another irony is that women who may have become involved with a career and less preoccupied with their inability to become pregnant had to take time from their work to undergo IVF treatment. They felt that they had to undertake IVF as a "duty" to attempt all possible routes to genetic parenthood for themselves and their husbands before they could accept a child-free life. Crowe concludes that like other technologies, IVF is not value-neutral, but

> . . . contains values in its design which reflect the social relations at the time of its innovation. IVF curtails any potential for the redefinition of parenthood — or infertility — by focusing exclusively on women's biological reproduction. In so doing it reinforces the notion of the "natural" bond between a mother and her biological children as well as reinforcing the idea that the nuclear family — or indeed one's own biological children — is the only desirable structure of social relations between adults and young children. (62)

Despite our culture's emphasis on motherhood, men are often the dominant partner in reproductive decisions. A study of 22 couples who were interviewed in a small city in New York State during 1985-86 found that reproductively normal husbands of infertile wives empathized with their wives' despair, but reproductively normal wives of infertile husbands considered themselves to be physiologically infertile as well (Greil et al. 1988). Involuntary childlessness is felt to be potentially discrediting, but male infertility is more damaging to masculinity than female infertility to femininity, and so fertile wives often protectively display a "courtesy stigma" (Miall 1985 and 1986). A study of voluntarily childless couples found that it was the husband's wishes that prevailed (Marciano 1978). When the wife wanted a child and the husband did not, they stayed childless; when the husband wanted a child and the wife did not, they often divorced. In interviews with women who terminated a pregnancy following a prenatal diagnosis of genetic or developmental defect, Rothman found it was the husbands who were sure about the decision to end the pregnancy, and who persuaded their wives of the wisdom of the decision (Rothman 1986).

In actuality, it is not that men *per se* control reproductive decisions, but that the dominant partner does, and in our society, the dominant partner is likely to be the man. Most of the couples in the research reported above were white. In the black community, where men do not have the generalized dominant status of white men, women are more likely to make the childbearing decisions. In interviews with black men in abortion waiting rooms, Shostak (1984: ch.5) found that the men who were especially resentful of their partners' decision to abort were those who ascribed to the cultural tenet that the man should be the boss, and who were traditionalists and wanted the continuance of the pregnancy. They were, says Shostak, ". . . doubly shocked: not only are they not to become fathers, but they are not to decide the matter, one way or the other."

In the light of such findings of male dominance in childbearing decisions, Rosen and Benson (1982:114) say that the assumption that the man is the second-class partner in parenting decisions reflects unexamined stereotypes. They say further, "Since the findings from a number of studies where the male was included in some way reveal considerable discrepancies between men's and women's reports of the same event, as well as the male dominance in most decision-making, it seems rather odd that researchers have continued to downplay the male's role." (Also see Bean et al. 1983; Bokemeier and Monroe, 1983; Monroe et al. 1985.)

The increasing popularity of the use of IVF treatment in cases of male infertility is understandable in the light of men's investment in biological parenting and women's willingness to take on the physiological responsibility for treatment (cf. Gilligan 1982). An early report from England of IVF treatment for low sperm count (oligospermia), low motility (asthenospermia) and abnormal morphology (teratospermia) in 41 couples with an average duration of infertility of 6.5 years had a very high success rate — 34% (Cohen et al. 1984). A subsequent communication from Australia was less positive, and warned that ". . . IVF patients experience greater anguish from failed fertilization than from the failure to achieve a pregnancy after embryo transfer" (Yovich 1984). The failure to fertilize a "good egg" is a male problem; the failure of a successfully fertilized embryo to implant in the womb is more likely to be perceived as a female problem. The comment suggests that physicians think that male infertility is more anguishing than female infertility. A pessimistic report from England on the results of IVF treatment in male infertility notes that if such treatment were successful, ". . . it would represent a major, and indeed the only advance in treatment for what seems at present the worst problem in infertility practice" (Hull and Glazener 1984). The use of IVF in male-factor infertility is now considered one of the most effective treatments, and ". . . opens up an area which will allow the treatment of a substantial population of infertile couples for whom before there was no effective treatment" (Yates and deKretser 1987, p. 145; Acosta 1987).

CONCLUSION

A study of couples who are about to undergo IVF treatment which includes a comparison of those with male and female infertility could shed much light on the social processes involved in the use of the new reproductive technology (Arditti 1985). It is assumed that religious, cultural, and family pressures influence the path to treatment, but much less is known about the bargaining and marital tradeoffs involved. One writer calls the technology "collaborative reproduction" (Robertson 1986), but also notes that all reproduction is collaborative. Extracorporeal conception exacerbates all of the tensions, conflicts, and potential for gender politics of sexual reproduction, both between the couple involved, and in the couple's interaction with the medical system.

I am not persuaded that the new reproductive technology makes women into victims, but I also do not think they are acting entirely autonomously. The dynamics of participation in such treatment illuminates issues of men's domination in reproduction and the extent to which women can truly control their bodies when faced with personal, psychological, familial, and community pressures to produce a biological child.

NOTE

1. The basic techniques of *in vitro* fertilization was established by Steptoe and Edwards (1978). The protocol requires a stimulation of ovulation with fertility drugs, removal of a viable egg or eggs using laparoscopy or ultrasound, fertilization of the ova with motile sperm in a petri dish (the "test tube"), incubation of the gametes until one or more multi-celled embryos is produced, and replacement of the embryo or embryos directly into the uterus through the vagina (Beier and

Lindner 1983; Crosignani 1983; Edwards and Purdy 1982; Edwards and Steptoe 1983; Hafez and Semm 1982; Hogden 1984; Jones et al. 1982; Lewin et al. 1986).

REFERENCES

Acosta, A. A., 1987. "The Role of IVF in Male Infertility." Presented at Fifth World Congress in *In Vitro* Fertilization and Embryo Transfer, Norfolk, VA.

Alder, E. and A. A. Templeton. 1985. "Patient Reaction to Treatment." *Lancet* 1(Jan. 19):168.

Andrews, L. B. 1984. *New Conceptions: A Consumer's Guide to the Newest Infertility Treatments*. New York: St. Martin's Press.

Appleton, T. 1986. "Caring for the IVF Patient—Counselling Care." Pp. 161-69 in *In Vitro Fertilization: Past, Present, Future*, edited by S. Fishel and E. M. Symonds. Oxford, IRL Press.

Aral, S. O. and W. Cates. 1983. "The Increasing Concern with Infertility: Why Now?" *Journal of the American Medical Association* 250:2327-31.

Arditti, R. 1985. "Reproductive Engineering and the Social Control of Women." *Radical America* 19:9-26.

Asch, R. H. et al. 1984. "Pregnancy After Translaparoscopic Gamete Intrafallopian Transfer." *Lancet* 2 (Nov. 3):1034-35.

Asch, R. H. et al. 1985. "Gamete Intrafallopian Transfer (GIFT): A New Treatment for Infertility." *International Journal of Fertility* 30:41-45.

Asch, R. H. et al. 1986a. "Preliminary Experiences with Gamete Intrafallopian Transfer (GIFT)," *Fertility and Sterility* 45:366-71.

Asch, R. H. et al. 1986b. "Gamete Intrafallopian Transfer (GIFT): Use of Minilaparotomy and an Individualized Regimen of Induction of Follicular Development." *Acta Europaea Fertilatatis* 17:187-193.

Bainbridge, I. 1982. "With Child in Mind: the Experiences of a Potential IVF Mother." Pp. 119-27 in *Test-Tube Babies*, edited by W.A.W. Walters and P. Singer. Melbourne: Oxford.

Bean, F. D. et al. 1983. "Husband-wife Communication, Wife's Employment and the Decision for Male or Female Sterilization." *Journal of Marriage and the Family* 45:395-403.

Beier, H. M. and H. R. Lindner (eds). 1983. *Fertilization of the Human Egg In Vitro*. Berlin: Springer-Verlag.

Bokemeier, J. L. and P. A. Monroe. 1983. "Continued Reliance on One Respondent in Family Decision-Making Studies: A Content Analysis." *Journal of Marriage and the Family* 45:645-52.

Brown, L. and J. Brown, with S. Freeman. 1979. *Our Miracle Called Louise*. London: Paddington Press.

Buster, J. E. et al. 1983. "Nonsurgical Transfer of *in Vivo* Fertilized Donated Ova to Five Infertile Women: Report of Two Pregnancies." *Lancet* 2(July 23):224-25.

Bustillo, M. et al. 1984. "Nonsurgical Ovum Transfer as a Treatment for Intractable Infertility: What Effectiveness Can We Realistically Expect?" *American Journal of Obstetrics and Gynecology* 148:(Mar. 1):508-12.

Calhoun, L. G. and J. W. Selby. 1980. "Voluntary Childlessness, Involuntary Childlessness, and Having Children: A Study of Social Perceptions." *Family Relations* 29:181-83.

Chico, N. P. and S. F. Hartley. 1981. "Widening Choices in Motherhood of the Future." *Psychology of Women Quarterly* 6:12-25.

Chodorow, N. 1978. *The Reproduction of Mothering.* Berkeley, CA: University of California Press.

Cohen, J. et al. 1984. "Male Infertility Successfully Treated by *in Vitro* Fertilization." *Lancet* 1(June 2):1238-39.

Cohen, J. et al. 1985. "*In Vitro* Fertilization: A Treatment for Male Infertility." *Fertility and Sterility* 43:422-32.

Cohen, J. et al. 1986. "Factors Affecting Survival and Implantation of Cryopreserved Human Embryos." *Journal of in Vitro Fertilization and Embryo Transfer* 3 (Feb.): 46-52.

Cohen, J., J. Hewitt and G. Rowland. 1984. "Application of *in Vitro* Fertilization in Cases of Poor Post-Coital Test." *Lancet* 2(Sept. 8):583.

Corea, G. 1985a. *The Mother Machine.* New York: Harper and Row.

Corea, G. 1985b. "IVF: A Game for Losers at Half of U.S. Clinics." *Medical Tribune.* July 3:1, 12-13.

Crosignani, P. G. 1983. *In Vitro Fertilization and Embryo Transfer.* London and New York: Academic Press.

Crowe, C. 1985. "'Women Want It': *In Vitro* Fertilization and Women's Motivations for Participation." *Women's Studies International Forum* 8:57-62.

Daniels, K. R. 1986. "New Birth Technologies—A Social Work Approach to Researching the Psychosocial Factors." *Social Work in Health Care* 11(4):49-60.

Editorial. 1937. "Conception in a Watch Glass." *New England Journal of Medicine* 109(Oct. 21):678.

Edwards, R. G. 1985. "*In Vitro* Fertilization and Embryo Replacement: Opening Lecture." *Annals of the New York Academy of Sciences* 442:1-22.

Edwards, R. G. and J. M. Purdy (eds.). 1982. *Human Conception in Vitro: Proceedings of the First Bourn Hall Meeting.* London and New York: Academic Press.

Edwards, R. G. and P. C. Steptoe. 1980. *A Matter of Life.* New York: Morrow.

Edwards, R. G. and P. C. Steptoe. 1983. "Current Status of *in Vitro* Fertilization and Implantation of Human Embryos." *Lancet* 2(Dec. 3):1265-69.

Fishel, S. 1986. "IVF—The Historical Perspective." Pp. 1-16 in *In Vitro Fertilization: Past, Present, Future,* edited by S. Fishel and E. M. Symonds. Oxford, IRL Press.

Fox, R. 1959. *Experiment Perilous.* Philadelphia: University of Pennsylvania Press.

Freeman, E. W. et al. 1985. "Psychological Evaluation and Support in a Program of *in Vitro* Fertilization and Embryo Transfer." *Fertility and Sterility* 43:48-53.

Freeman, L., A. Trounson, and C. Kirby, 1986. "Cryopreservation of Human Embryos: Progress on the Clinical Use of the Technique in Human *in Vitro* Fertilization." *Journal of in Vitro Fertilization and Embryo Transfer* 3(Feb.): 53-61.

Gilligan, C. 1982. *In a Different Voice*. Cambridge, MA: Harvard.

Given, J. E., G. S. Jones and D. L. McMillen. 1985. "A Comparison of Personality Characteristics between *in Vitro* Fertilization Patients and Other Infertile Patients." *Journal of in Vitro Fertilization and Embryo Transfer* 2:49-54.

Gorovitz, S. 1985. "Engineering Human Reproduction: A Challenge to Public Policy." *Journal of Medicine and Philosophy* 10:267-74.

Greenfeld, D. et al. 1985. "The Role of the Social Worker in the *In Vitro* Fertilization Program." *Social Work in Health Care* 10:71-79.

Greenfield, D., M. P. Diamond and A. H. DeCherney. 1987. "Grief Reactions Following *In Vitro* Fertilization Treatment." *Journal of Psychosomatic Ob/ Gyn* (in press).

Greil, A. L., T. A. Leitko, and K. L. Porter. 1988. "Infertility: His and Hers." Gender & Society 2:forthcoming.

Hafez, E. S. E. and K. Semm (eds.). 1982. *In Vitro Fertilization and Embryo Transfer*. New York: Alan R. Liss.

Harris, M. 1986. "Caring for the IVF Patient—Nursing Care." Pp. 155-160 in *In Vitro Fertilization: Past, Present, Future*, edited by S. Fishel and E. M. Symonds. Oxford, IRL Press.

Haseltine, F. P. et al. 1985. "Psychological Interviews in Screening Couples Undergoing *in Vitro* Fertilization." *Annals of the New York Academy of Sciences* 442:504-22.

Hatch, M. 1984. "Mother, Father, Worker: Men and Women and Reproductive Risks of Work." Pp. 161-79 in *Double Exposure*, edited by W. Chavkin. New York: Monthly Review Press.

Haug, M. and Lavin, B. 1983. *Consumerism in Medicine*. Beverly Hills, CA: Sage Publications.

Henley, J. A. 1982. "IVF and the Human Family: Possible and Likely Consequences." Pp. 79-87 in *Test-Tube Babies*, edited by W.A.W. Walters and P. Singer. Melbourne: Oxford.

Hewitt, J. et al. 1985. "Treatment of Idiopathic Infertility, Cervical Mucus Hostility, and Male Infertility: Artificial Insemination with Husband's Semen or *in Vitro* Fertilization?" *Fertility and Sterility* 44:350-55.

Hirsch, I. et al. 1985. "*In Vitro* Fertilization in Couples with Male Factor Infertility." *Fertility and Sterility* 45:659-64.

Hogden, G. D. 1984. "Summary of Current Status of *in Vitro* Fertilization and Embryo Transfer Therapy." Presented at Third World Congress on *In Vitro* Fertilization and Embryo Transfer, Helsinki.

Hubbard, R. 1981. "The Case Against *in Vitro* Fertilization and Implantation."

Pp. 159-62 in *The Custom-Made Child*, edited by H. B. Holmes, B. B. Hoskins, and M. Gross. Clifton, NJ: Humana Press.

Hull, M. G. R. and C. M. A. Glazener. 1984. "Male Infertility and *in Vitro* Fertilization." *Lancet* 2(July 28):231.

Hull, M. G. R. et al. 1985a. "Population Study of Causes, Treatment, and Outcome of Infertility." *British Medical Journal* 291(Dec. 14):1693-97.

Hull, M. G. R. et al. 1985b. "An Economic and Ethical Way to Introduce *in Vitro* Fertilization to Infertility Practice, and Findings Related to Postcoital Sperm/Mucus Penetration in Isolated Tubal, 'Cervical,' and Unexplained Infertility." *Annals of New York Academy of Sciences* 442:318-23.

Jarrell, J. et al. 1986. "An *in Vitro* Fertilization and Embryo Transfer Pilot Study: Treatment-Dependent and Treatment-Independent Pregnancies." *American Journal of Obstetrics and Gynecology* 154:231-35.

Johnston, W. I. H. et al. 1985. "Patient Selection for *in Vitro* Fertilization." *Annals of the New York Academy of Sciences* 442:523-32.

Jones, H. W. et al. 1982. "The Program for *in Vitro* Fertilization at Norfolk." *Fertility and Society* 38:14-21.

Jones, H. W. 1986. "The Infertile Couple." Pp. 17-26 in *In Vitro Fertilization: Past, Present, Future*, edited by S. Fishel and E. M. Symonds. Oxford, IRL Press.

Kemeter, P., A. Eder, and M. Springer-Kremser. 1985. "Psychosocial Testing and Pretreatment of Women for *in Vitro* Fertilization." *Annals of the New York Academy of Sciences* 442:490-503.

Kemeter, P. et al. 1986. "*In Vitro* Fertilization Patients and the Outcome of *in Vitro* Fertilization: Psychosocial and Psychoendocrinological Factors." Pp. 89-101 in *Research in Psychosomatic Obstetrics and Gynaecology*, edited by B. Leysen, P. Nijs and D. Richter. Leuven: Acco.

Kolata, G. 1983. "*In Vitro* Fertilization Goes Commercial." *Science* 221(Sept. 16):1160-61.

Leeton, J. and J. Harman. 1986. "Attitudes Toward Egg Donation of Thirty-Four Infertile Women Who Donated During Their *in Vitro* Fertilization Treatment." *Journal of in Vitro Fertilization and Embryo Transfer* 3:374-78.

Leeton, J., A. O. Trounson, and C. Wood. 1982. "IVF and ET: What It Is and How It Works." Pp. 2-10 in *Test-Tube Babies*, edited by W. Walters and P. Singer. Melbourne: Oxford.

Leeton, J. et al. 1984. "Unexplained Infertility and the Possibilities of Management with *in Vitro* Fertilization and Embryo Transfer." *Australia/New Zealand Journal of Obstetrics and Gynecology* 24:131-34.

Leeton, J. et al. 1986. "Pregnancy Established in an Infertile Patient After Transfer of an Embryo Fertilized *in Vitro* Where the Oocyte was Donated by the Sister of the Recipient." *Journal of in Vitro Fertilization and Embryo Transfer* 3:379-82.

Leitko, T. A. and A. L. Greil. 1985. "Gender, Involuntary Childlessness and Emotional Distress." Presented at Annual Meetings, American Sociological Association, Washington, DC.

Lewin, A. et al. 1986. "Ultrasonically Guided Oocyte Recovery for *in Vitro* Fertilization: An Improved Method." *Journal of in Vitro Fertilization and Embryo Transfer* 3:370-73.

Lizza, E. F. et al. 1984. "Advances in Diagnosis and Treatment of Male Infertility." *West Virginia Medical Journal* 80:45-50.

Mahadevan, M. M. et al. 1985. "Successful Use of *in Vitro* Fertilization with Persisting Low-Quality Semen." *Annals of the New York Academy of Sciences* 442:293-30.

Mahlstedt, P. P. 1985. "The Psychological Component of Infertility." *Fertility and Sterility* 43:335-46.

Mahlstedt, P. P. and S. Macduff. 1985. "Emotional Factors and the IVF-ET Process." Presented at the Annual Meeting, American Fertility Society, Chicago.

Marciano, T. D. 1978. "Male Pressure in the Decision to Remain Childfree." *Alternative Lifestyles* 1:95-111.

Matthews, R. and A. M. Matthews. 1986. "Infertility and Involuntary Childlessness: The Transition to Nonparenthood." *Journal of Marriage and the Family* 48:641-49.

Mazor, M. D. 1984. "Emotional Reactions to Infertility." Pp. 23-35 in *Infertility: Medical, Emotional and Social Considerations*, edited by M. D. Mazor and H. F. Simons. New York: Human Sciences Press.

Mazor, M. D. and H. F. Simons (eds.). 1984. *Infertility: Medical, Emotional and Social Considerations*. New York: Human Sciences Press.

Mazure, C. et al. 1985. "Analysis of Psychological Data in 97 IVF Couples." Presented at Annual Meeting, American Fertility Society, Chicago.

Menning, B. E. 1977. *Infertility: A Guide for the Childless Couple*. Englewood Cliffs, NJ: Prentice-Hall.

Menning, B. E. 1982. "The Psychosocial Impact of Infertility." *Nursing Clinics of North America* 17:155-63.

Miall, C. E. 1985. "Perceptions of Informal Sanctioning and the Stigma of Involuntary Childlessness." *Deviant Behavior* 6:383-403.

Miall, C. E. 1986. "The Stigma of Involuntary Childlessness." *Social Problems* 33:268-82.

Mikesell, S. G. and R. Falk. 1985. "Low Marital Distress Reported by *In Vitro* Fertilization Participants." Presented at Annual Meeting, American Fertility Society, Chicago.

Mishler, E. G. 1984. *The Discourse of Medicine: Dialectics of Medical Interviews*. Norwood, NJ: Ablex.

Monroe, A. et al. 1985. "Spousal Response Consistency in Decision-Making Research." *Journal of Marriage and the Family* 47:733-38.

Mushin, D. N., M. C. Berreda-Hanson, and J. C. Spensley. 1986. "*In Vitro* Fertilization Children: Early Psychosocial Development." *Journal of in Vitro Fertilization and Embryo Transfer* 3(Aug.):247-52.

Robertson, J. A. 1986. "Embryos, Families, and Procreative Liberty: The Legal

Structure of the New Reproduction." *Southern California Law Review* 59(July):939-1041.

Rogers, P. A. W. and A. O. Trounson. 1986. "IVF: The Future." Pp. 229-45 in *In Vitro Fertilization: Past, Present, Future*, edited by S. Fishel and E. M. Symonds. Oxford, IRL Press.

Rosen, R. H. and T. Benson. 1982. "The Second-Class Partner: The Male Role in Family-Planning Decisions." Pp. 97-124 in *The Child Bearing Decision*, edited by G. L. Fox. Beverly Hills, CA: Sage.

Rosenwaks, Z., L. L. Veeck and H. Liu. 1986. "Pregnancy Following Transfer of *in Vitro* Fertilized Donated Oocytes." *Fertility and Sterility* 45:417-20.

Ross, L. S. 1983. "Diagnosis and Treatment of Infertile Men: A Clinical Perspective." *Journal of Urology* 130:847-54.

Rossi, A. S. 1977. "A Biosocial Perspective on Parenting." *Daedalus* 106:1-31.

Rossi, A. S. 1984. "Gender and Parenthood." *American Sociological Review* 49:1-19.

Rothman, B. K. 1984. "The Meanings of Choice in Reproductive Technology." Pp. 22-33 in *Test-Tube Women*, edited by R. Arditti, R. Duelli-Klein, and S. Minden. London: Pandora.

Rothman, B. K. 1986. *The Tentative Pregnancy*. New York: Viking.

Rudkin, D. 1977. *Ashes*. Berkeley, CA: West Coast Plays.

Saunders, D. M., M. Mathews, and P. A. L. Lancaster. 1987. "The Australian Register, Current Research and Future Role. (A Preliminary Report)." Presented at Fifth World Congress on *In Vitro* Fertilization and Embryo Transfer, Norfolk, VA.

Seppala, M. 1985. "The World Collaborative Report on *in Vitro* Fertilization and Embryo Replacement: Current State of the Art in January 1984." *Annals of the New York Academy of Sciences*. 442:558-63.

Sher, G. et al. 1983. "*In Vitro* Sperm Capacitation and Transcervical Intrauterine Insemination for the Treatment of Refractory Infertility: Phase I." *Fertility and Sterility* 41:260-64.

Shostak, A. B. and G. Mclouth. 1984. *Men and Abortion*. New York: Praeger.

Shrednick, A. 1983. "Emotional Support Programs for *in Vitro* Fertilization." *Fertility and Sterility* 40:704.

Singer, P. and D. Wells. 1985. *Making Babies: The New Science and Ethics of Conception*. New York: Scribner.

Soules, M. R. 1985. "The *in Vitro* Fertilization Pregnancy Rate: Let's Be Honest With One Another." *Fertility and Sterility* 43:511-13.

Steptoe, P. C. and R. G. Edwards. 1978. "Birth After Reimplantation of a Human Embryo." *Lancet* 2(Aug. 12): 366.

Trotsky, L. 1925. Address to the Third All-Union Conference on Protection of Mothers and Children. *Pravda*, Dec. 7. Cited in G. W. Lapidus. 1978. *Women in Soviet Society*. Berkeley: University of California Press, at p. 81.

Trounson, A. et al. 1983. "Pregnancy Established in an Infertile Patient After Transfer of a Donated Embryo Fertilized *in Vitro*." *British Medical Journal* 286(Mar. 12):835-38.

Waitzkin, H. 1983. *The Second Sickness: Contradictions of Capitalist Health Care*. New York: Free Press.

Walters, W. A. W. and P. Singer (eds.). 1982. *Test-Tube Babies*. Melbourne: Oxford.

Wood, C. and A. Westmore. 1984. *Test-Tube Conception*. Englewood Cliffs, NJ: Prentice-Hall.

Yates, C. A. and D. M. deKretser. 1987. "Male-Factor Infertility and *In Vitro* Fertilization." *Journal of In Vitro Fertilization and Embryo Transfer* 4:141-147.

Yovich, J. L., J. D. Stanger, and J. M. Yovich. 1985. "The Management of Oligospermia Infertility in *in Vitro* Fertilization." *Annals of the New York Academy of Sciences* 442:276-86.

Yovich, J. L., et al. 1986. "Developmental Assessment of Twenty *in Vitro* Fertilization (IVF) Infants at Their First Birthday." *Journal of in Vitro Fertilization and Embryo Transfer* 3(Aug.):253-57.

A Womb of His Own

Elaine Hoffman Baruch

SUMMARY. Although some feminists formerly saw utopian possibilities in reproductive technology, many now fear that the new technologies are turning women's bodies into test tubes. They feel that these technologies are designed less to help infertile women than to appease men's envy of women's reproductive power. The consequences of the new technologies for the psychology of women and children and the future creation of culture are open questions. Should the technologies succeed in taking reproduction out of the body altogether, it remains to be seen whether women will gain in freedom, or whether this will simply fulfill the age-old misogynistic fantasy of depriving women of their central place in procreation.

The women's movement began in part as a protest against forced labor—men's appropriation of women's bodies for reproduction. In 1970, Shulamith Firestone's *Dialectic of Sex*, a germinal book for the movement, proclaimed as part of a revolutionary manifesto that only by taking reproduction out of the body could women be free. In a transvaluation of Huxley's *Brave New World*, Firestone argued that freedom for women meant freedom from reproductive biology. A number of feminist utopian writers argued similarly. In 1976, Marge Piercy, for example, in her extraordinary vision of the future, *Woman on the Edge of Time*, which was a kind of bible for many feminists, claimed that only by women giving up their old power, that of reproduction, could equality of the sexes be achieved. The individuals in her utopia reproduce themselves in a charming prenatal nursery where unborn "babies"—if one can call them that—joggle together happily in a kind of giant aquarium.[1] No isolated test tubes for them.

But now that reproduction *ex utero* is less of a sci-fi fantasy than

135

formerly, many feminists fear that women will soon have to fight for the right to have children in the "natural" way at all. It is not just "test-tube babies" that we have to be concerned with. Rather as one book puts it, it is "test-tube women" that should engage our attention. The "medocrats," those doctors in love with their new technological toys — are turning the bodies of women themselves into test tubes, where they conduct their ill-conceived experiments.[2]

Given these premises, it is easy to have a scenario of gloom follow. The scientist is seen as a type of contemporary Frankenstein, who snatches the eggs out of a woman's body in his attempt to recreate life. If in the past, men deprived woman of a public space, now they plunder her inner space, so that she no longer has a womb of her own.

Control over one's own body is perhaps the central feminist credo. It is what is now feared will be lost through the new technology. It was perhaps inevitable in our technological age that conception, the last of the cottage industries, would be taken out of the home and placed in the antiseptic factory of the lab. The fear is that all reproduction will become artificial, given the technical means for it, and that contrary to Shulamith Firestone's belief, which assumed good intentions in a post-revolutionary society, reproductive technology in patriarchy is not good for women.

One might argue that *in vitro* fertilization and surrogate motherhood can alleviate the pain of infertility. But one might then counter that much of that pain has been socially constructed. Why the necessity to have one's *own* child? And given that seemingly central value in patriarchal society, what is the place of the surrogate mother who is not bearing her own child — or rather *is* bearing her own child for others, for she is not a surrogate at all, but a real mother? (The term *surrogate* is a misnomer that we should be thinking of changing now although it is probably already too late.)[3]

No doubt the prospect of using surrogates will please men who wish to have children but want nothing to do with the mothers of their children. Surrogacy gives a man the opportunity to buy a womb of his own, without any concern for the woman to whom it is attached. The possibilities for exploitation of economically deprived women for surrogacy, both here and in the third world, whether by married or single men, are great. But the recommendation of the Warnock Committee in Great Britain that commercial surrogacy be a criminal offense might lead to even more exploitation—certainly to less freedom of reproductive choice. If a woman wishes to work in this way, why *should* her labor be free? But would the child born of surrogacy feel as if he had a womb of his own instead of a mother, particularly if he were the child of a single man?

A child can now have three "mothers": a genetic mother who supplies the ovum, a gestational mother who supplies the uterine environment, and a nurturing mother who provides the postnatal care.

What are the implications of these new possibilities for the psychology of the individual? Will the problems of identity felt by an adopted child be increased in the child who has three mothers, or will she feel more loved, particularly if all three mothers continue a relationship with her—not a common procedure right now. And what of the three mothers themselves? What are their rights? Their needs? Can they be sure they know what they will feel before undertaking the journey of communal, if sequential, parenting. Even this question assumes that they had a real choice to begin with and were not forced into arrangements by economic or emotional need.

To push the plot lines further, some day it may be possible for a child to have no mother at all, that is, for reproduction to take place completely outside the body. What will be the consequences for the development of the individual? The psychoanalyst Melanie Klein believes that all religion and art, all the achievements of culture, perhaps, are attempts to recover the mother's body symbolically.[4] What consequences would reproduction *ex utero* have on the relation of the individual to nature, art, other people, the world at large? Of course, it is possible for a child to be created *ex utero* and still have a nurturing mother. Marge Piercy gives all of her artificially created children three mothers, some of whom, by the way, are men. Under such conditions would there still be attempts to recapture symbolically the nurturing mother or mothers of one's childhood? And what would happen to women in a world without pregnancy? Would they gain freedom as in Piercy's vision, or would they be even less valued than they are now?

Misogynists from the ancient Hebrews and the Greeks have

dreamt of different ways of making babies — ways that would eliminate women. What else is the story of the creation of Eve about, at
least in the rib version, or the myth of Athena springing from the
head of Zeus — or of Dionysus coming out of his thigh? In the
Eumenides, Aeschylus's fifth century B.C. play, woman is spoken
of as a mere incubator; the real parent is the father. Both Jason in
Euripides' *Medea* and Hippolytus, in his play of the same name,
dream of a world in which babies will be created without those
difficult creatures — women. Fatherhood — without motherhood —
has been the desire behind these fantasies. It is a common belief
among feminists now that the new technology with its *in vitro* fertilization and embryo transfer was designed less to help the infertile
than to appease men's envy of women's reproductive power. Once
again, womb envy, as Karen Horney calls it, rears its ugly head. It
is no small surprise to find that on the issue of reproductive technology, some radical feminists sound more like the women of the New
Right than anyone else. They too fear men's intrusion into motherhood, the *sanctum sanctorum*.

There are some differences, however. Many of the same feminists who fear replacement of the mother have no objection to making woman the sole parent through parthenogenesis, which, should
it be achieved in humans, would produce only female children.
Both sexes have fantasies of omnipotence, it seems. Perhaps rather
than condemn the technology, both sexes should have equal opportunity to use it in order to realize their fantasies of sole parenting.
Or perhaps reproductive technology should not be used to gratify
either sex's narcissism. Besides it is more likely that men alone
would have access to the technology. At least that is one of the great
fears of women.

But in the feminist attack on technology as male conspiracy,
there is little recognition of the part that technology has had in
women's liberation, through contraception, abortion and the use of
machines in place of muscles; or the place it might have in future
liberation, through modifying biology, by lengthening the childbearing years for example, for those women who want that possibility.

There are reasons for the fears. Changes are accelerating at virtu-
oso speed with seemingly little participation by women. As Ama-

deo D'Adamo and I have said elsewhere, "Rather than be its passive recipients, women must become actively involved in determining the development and values of reproductive technology to end or at least mitigate the male domination of reproduction."[5]

NOTES

1. See *Women in Search of Utopia*, eds. Ruby Rohrlich and Elaine Hoffman Baruch (New York: Schocken Books, 1984), for a discussion of these works.

2. *Test-Tube Women: What Future for Motherhood?* Eds. Rita Arditti, Renate Duelli Klein, Shelley Minden (Boston: Pandora Press, 1984).

3. Some "surrogate" mothers advocate using the term "birth mother." However, new terms are needed to indicate the differences between the woman who contributes the oocyte, and the woman who gestates the embryo. They do not necessarily have to be the same woman.

4. See, for example, *Love, Hate, and Reparation* (New York: Norton, 1964).

5. "Resetting the Biological Clock: Women and the New Reproductive Technologies," *Dissent*, Summer, 1985.

Psychological Effects of
the New Reproductive Technologies

Eleanor Schuker

SUMMARY. Four psychological principles help us to understand the psychological effects of the new technologies: (1) Special circumstances of parenting and birth will stimulate fantasies in parents and children, which in turn influence the child's personality and identity; (2) Human parenting does not require a biological connection; nonbiological parents can be equally effective nurturers; (3) Good parenting involves a psychological interaction beginning at birth, so that early and permanent opportunity for attachment is important for normal development; (4) New technologies relieve the psychological pain of infertility and provide benefit by giving some individuals the opportunity to be parents. The psychology of surrogate mothers is also discussed.

Parenting is a challenging life task. It is no easy job to help a child of any given endowment to grow into a healthy mature personality. The new reproductive technologies have the potential to significantly affect both the psychological development of individuals who are the products of these technologies and the psychological attitudes of parents who use these vehicles. I will discuss four basic psychological principles which will help us to understand these potential effects.

The first principle is that a specific circumstance of birth or parenting will inevitably be given psychological meaning. Parents and

---

At the time of reediting this manuscript, the Stern-Whitehead "Baby M" surrogate mother case has just begun. It well-illustrates some of these dilemmas. Baby M's need is for firm continuous placement with a single set of psychologically stable parents.

children can create myths, elaborate in fantasy, and ascribe emotional significance to these circumstances of birth, as they are comprehended. Human imagination is wide-ranging and reflects individual needs, hopes, fears, and distortions. We might understand some possible psychological effects of atypical circumstances of birth or parenting by looking at the nature of fantasies and attitudes which can develop in a similar situation, that of adoption. Here the psychoanalytic literature is useful (Blum 1983, Brinich 1980 and 1982, Schechter 1967). A child learns of its adoption through ways it is treated, implicit and covert messages, and direct telling. It reacts in ways that depend on age, the developmental issues with which it is coping and the meanings (both conscious and unconscious) that parents transmit. Having two sets of parents, biological and nurturant, can stimulate a child's fantasy that it has been specially chosen (influencing character in either a positive or pathological direction). Or a child can feel that it has been abandoned or is worthy of (re-)abandonment. Using primitive thinking characteristic of small children, the child may split parental sets into "all-good" and "all-bad," and retain a hope of finding the idealized good parent. Identity issues can be complicated by these fantasies, as well as by an atmosphere of family secrets which interferes with a firm sense of who one is. The shrouding of circumstances of birth in secrecy or untruths can be a part of family patterns of withholding, dishonesty, or shame. An adoptive parent can help a child to come to terms with the realistic facts of its birth in a healthy way if the parent is at peace with the realities. However, the adoptive parent may also need to see the child as a repair for a damaged self, or for an incompletely mourned narcissistic wound of infertility. The child can be overvalued, or can be seen as a disappointment. A parent can also see an adoptive child as a "bad seed," imperfect, or as a rejected part of him/herself which is then disavowed.

All parents and children have fantasies, conflicts, and problems. However, the unusual circumstance of birth can become an important focus for fantasies or conflicts. Thus these birth circumstances may be an important theme in the personality, without necessarily implying greater pathology. We would expect this to be the case for those individuals who are products of the new technologies. The unconscious and conscious meanings of these circumstances, as conveyed by parents and reshaped in the child's growing fantasies, will affect the child's self-image.

A major question raised by the new reproductive technologies is whether there is a relation between biological connection and adequacy of parenting. The second psychological principle is that parenting in humans does not require or depend on a biological connection. A nonbiological parent can be as effective as a biological parent. This is because much of human attachment and relatedness depends on social, environmental, or internal mental (fantasy) life, rather than on reflex or instinctual biology. Capacity for motherliness is dependent on the personality of the woman, her own experiences with being nurtured as a child, plus her current emotional support and her investment in or commitment to parenting. Biological connections play a role only to the degree that these connections have psychological meaning to that individual. For example, parents or grandparents may act in a rejecting way to a nonbiological child if it does not have some desired familial characteristic (Blum 1983). Of course, biological parents can reject a child for similar psychodynamic reasons, also. Some women may feel inadequate and therefore have difficulties attaching to a child if they have not experienced pregnancy, but this is by no means the rule for adoptive mothers. In cultures where parenting by nonbiological parents is normative and expected, the parent is likely to be less conflicted. We do know quite a bit about how the capacity for maternal behavior develops in humans, and it is a psychological process. The rudiments of maternal behavior are evident in a little girl by the second and third year of life (Galenson 1981; Kleeman 1976), and grow in intimate connection with her gender identity, her learned awareness of her reproductive potential and her gender role, and her early identifications. Maternalism is further reinforced as she grows to adolescence and adulthood (Blum 1976; Kestenberg 1976) and may be enhanced by cultural influences and an experience of pregnancy or child-caretaking. Capacities for nurturant and paternal behavior are also developed from early life in boys, though somewhat differently (Ross 1977). Numerous studies have shown that individuals with deficient early mothering experiences have deficits in parenting capacity as adults (Spitz 1965). Thus the key factor in adequate parenting performance is the experience of being well-nurtured oneself.

The third psychological principle is that the process of parenting involves an interaction between parent and child which starts from birth. A bond is formed through the many physical, social and emotional interactions that occur in the course of caretaking and play activities between parent and child from earliest life. The parents' capacities to attune to the child's needs and the child's endowment facilitate a growing bond in both parties. Significant psychological developmental processes occur in the earliest weeks and months of life that profoundly affect the child's development (Spitz 1965; Stern 1985; Beebe 1982; Greenspan 1981). Thus, early disruptions in attachment, delay in assignment, prolonged separations from the nurturant parents, or parental uncertainty about the firmness and permanency of the attachment can all have serious damaging effects on the child's development. Legal uncertainties related to the new technologies run the risk of delaying or disrupting placement, thus interfering with normal psychological development and with the attachment processes in both parents and child. The fact that adoptive parents (or parents who raise a child conceived by surrogate motherhood or artificial insemination) can be highly successful nurturers illustrates the centrality of psychological, not biological connectedness.

It may be useful to add a brief comment here about the psychology of surrogate mothers, to clarify some of the psychological issues which should be considered before making legal decisions about this process. There are a few published psychological studies of surrogate mothers which have involved psychiatric interviewing (Franks 1981; Parker 1984). My own work has involved in-depth psychoanalytic interviews with a few surrogates, including eliciting dream material, as a way of trying to understand fantasies and motivations in surrogates (Schuker). Often surrogate mothers had altruistic and idealistic feelings about giving a "gift" of a child to an infertile couple. The surrogate may have been close to an infertile woman, and known her pain. The surrogate often had enjoyed previous pregnancies, and felt that being pregnant was something she could do well, an achievement. There was less pleasure and investment in the task of raising children itself for some of these women. Contrary to some common beliefs, financial gain does not seem to be a prime motivation for most surrogate mothers, though there may be a secondary need for some assistance to substitute for other employment. I have been impressed by the strong wish to give this "special gift" as a way of becoming special. One woman told me: "I'm an ordinary person. I really don't have special talents. But being pregnant is something I do well. This is something I could do that would be very special." She fantasied and dreamed that the parental couple would be forever grateful to her. Some surrogate mothers are also motivated by a wish to repair a previous experience, such as an abortion or relinquishment of a baby for adoption, and now fantasize a reparative controlled placement. The surrogate may need to grieve for the loss of the fetus/baby and whatever its particular meaning to her, and the handling of the post-birth experience by those around her may be crucial to her self-esteem.

A fourth psychological principle is important to mention in evaluating the new technologies, though it may seem obvious. Medical research is involved in new technologies in the hope of eliminating infertility and relieving the psychological pain and stress of that condition.

Having discussed these four basic psychological principles, I want to mention some other issues raised by the new technologies of reproduction. My personal bias is toward minimizing social controls and maximizing voluntary choice in the application of these technologies. This is because I fear that advocates of social controls over others' decisions about their bodies and lives tend to be expressing their own prejudices and deep psychological needs and their own wishes to dominate and control others for their own purposes. An individual who wants to try to solve a personal medical problem, or to improve his/her own genetic line through new technologies is less likely to be dangerous to human freedom than someone who wants to impose his/her views of genetic or behavioral perfection on someone else. Another issue is raised about the consequences of the potential for new technologies to reset the "biological clock," enabling women to be mothers at a different time in their lives. Will this affect mothering capacities? Can a woman whose frozen embryos were harvested previously, then grown in a gestational mother, perhaps after fertilization *in vitro*, make an effective psychological parent? My answer is that the technological facts do not rule out the woman's capacity to be an excellent parent. Her capacity for mothering is a psychological issue, perhaps better understood by examining the meanings of these particular choices. Similarly a young teenager's capacity to achieve biological parenthood is not a useful indicator of either her capacity for nurturing behavior or even her psychological readiness to parent. Whether the woman is older or younger, I feel that each individual must make the choice about her commitment to be a parent. Ideally she will make this choice in an environment that provides educational information, psychological support, and the best available medical skills.

BIBLIOGRAPHY

Annas, G. 1984. "Redefining Parenthood. . . . " *Hastings Report* 14(5):50-52.

Baruch, E. H. and A. F. D'Adamo, Jr. 1985. "Resetting the Biological Clock." *Dissent* Summer:273-276.

Beebe, B. et al. 1982. "Assessment and Treatment of Mother-Infant Attunement." *Psychoanalytic Inquiry* 1:601-623.

Berger, D. M. 1980. "Reactions to Male Infertility." *American Journal of Psychiatry* 137, 9:1047 ff.

Blum, H. P. 1976. "Masochism, Ego Ideal, and the Psychology of Women." *Journal of the American Psychoanalytic Association* 24,5: 157-192.

Blum, H. P. 1983. "Adoptive Parents: Generative Conflict." *Psychoanalytic Study of the Child* 38:141-164.

Brinich, P. 1980. "Potential Effects of Adoption on the Self and Object Relationships." *Psychoanalytic Study of the Child* 35:107-134.

Brinich, P. et al. 1982. "Adoption and Adaptation." *Journal of Nervous and Mental Diseases* 170:489-493.

Freeman, E. et al. 1985. "Psychological Evaluation and Support before IVF-ET." *Fertility and Sterility* 43(Jan.):48-53.

Franks, P. D., 1981. "Psychological Evaluation of . . . Surrogate Mother Programs." *American Journal of Psychiatry* 138:1378-9.

Galenson, E. and H. Roiphe. 1981. *Infantile Origins of Sexual Identity*. New York: International Universities Press.

Greenspan, S. I. 1981. *Psychopathology and Adaptation in Infancy and Early Childhood*. New York: International Universities Press.

Kestenberg, J. 1976. "Regression and Reintegration in Pregnancy." *Journal of the American Psychoanalytic Association*. 24:213-251.

Kleeman, J. A. 1976. "Freud's Views on Early Female Sexuality in Light of Direct Child Observation." *Journal of the American Psychoanalytic Association*. 24:3-28.

Parker, P. J. 1984. "Surrogate Motherhood . . . Psch. Screening." *Bulletin of the American Academy of Psychiatry and the Law* 12:21-39.

Ross, J. M. 1977. "Toward Fatherhood: The Epigenesis of Paternal Identity." *International Journal of Psychoanalysis* 60:327-347.

Schechter, M. D. 1967. *Panel: Psychoanalytic Theory as it Relates to Adoption*. *Journal of the American Psychoanalytic Association*. 15:695-708.

Schuker, E. Unpublished data.

Spitz, R. 1965. *The First Year of Life*. New York: International Universities Press.

Stern, D. M. 1985. *The Interpersonal World of the Infant*. New York: Basic Books.

Brave New Baby
in the Brave New World

Betty Jean Lifton

SUMMARY. Society would be wise to ponder the psychology of
the adopted in order to gain some insights into what the psychological makeup of the brave new baby might be. Whatever combinations
of reproduction and parenting we make, we should relinquish the
secrecy that has been the scourge of the adoption system.

I do want to make one confession: until I read about all of this
wonderful new technology, I had thought of adopted people as very
exotic. We are related to Oedipus: we belong to myth. But our
brave new babies make the adopted seem *passé*. Oedipus, after all,
was conceived in an old fashioned human scenario which involved
physical love (despite the inhuman behavior of his parents after his
birth.)

Yet, society would be wise to ponder the psychology of the
adopted in order to gain some insights into what might be the psychological makeup of our brave new babies. They have much in
common. The adoptee is a genetic stranger accepted into a biologi-

---

As an adoptee, I am very glad to have been chosen (adoptees are always chosen
and expected to be grateful) to present here the rights of the embryo, or, I should
say, the rights of the brave new embryo who is going to become the brave new
baby. In the past, I might point out, the old embryos and babies had little or no
rights in spite of that oft heard phrase "in the best interest of the child." The best
interests of the child always come down to the best interests of the adults involved. In this case, we are referring to the adults who hope to benefit from the
new reproductive technology that is tampering with a birth process that until
now—when you consider the overpopulation of the world—Nature has been handling quite well.

149

cally unrelated family *as if* actually related; in other worlds, the adoptee is a product of social engineering. Our brave new baby may be genetically related to one or both parents, but will be raised *as if* born to both in a natural way; in fact, the baby is a product of scientific engineering. Both adoptee and new baby will share the perilous *as if* factor, with its destructive by-product: secrecy. Secrecy, as the adoptee knows well, produces a feeling of isolation and despair in the very person whom it is meant to protect.

As I have written previously, the adoptee, by being extruded from his or her own biological clan, forced out of the natural flow of generational continuity, feels forced out of nature itself. The adoptee feels an alien, an outsider, an orphan, a foundling, a changeling—outside the natural realm of being. I suggest that the brave new baby, whether created *in vitro* by embryo transfer or by a surrogate mother, will feel the same sense of alienation and bewilderment upon learning the unnatural ways she or he came into the world. The absence of some part of one's heritage is always felt.

Psychological studies of the adopted have revealed that it is hard to build a sense of self when one is raised in secrecy, when the truth about oneself is distorted or hidden. Psychiatrists have found that adopted children who are confused about their origins suffer from "genealogical bewilderment" (not understanding where one comes from) and "adoption stress" (not being able to cope with the confusion). They are insecure and maladjusted. Clinics and residential treatment centers have been reporting seeing a disproportionate number of adopted children.

There will be new terms for what our brave new babies will suffer from—shall we say "technological bewilderment" and "conception stress." Their confusion may well result in many of the symptoms seen in some adoptees: low self-esteem, lack of trust and a preoccupation with fantasy.

On the positive side, the new baby has advantages the adoptee does not: genetic relatedness to at least one parent, if not two, and historical continuity with the biological clan. But studies have shown that lack of knowledge about even one parent can be as damaging as lack of knowledge about both—and many new babies will have only one known parent.

Like adoptees, these new babies will be assured how much they were wanted, how much superior they are to a blood related baby or a baby conceived in a natural way. But also like adoptees, they will have secrets of their own: they will know that rather than having been first choice, they were second best to the child who might have been had their parents been able to have children in the natural way.

I keep trying to imagine what will happen when this brave new baby asks, as Oedipus did, "Who am I?" There will be no oracle to consult, no Tiresias to issue dire warnings, no social workers to discourage him. Instead the brave new baby will have to seek scientists in laboratories, doctors with turkey syringes, lawyers with legal briefs. Like the adoptee, the brave new baby will find that the truth of her or his missing origins are sealed: perhaps in a sperm bank, or, if born of a surrogate, in the vital statistics archive where the original birth certificates of adoptees molder away. It is possible — and this is the most tragic — that false names may have been given or records not kept.

Other questions will surface after the brave new baby utters the first "Who Am I?" Who is my real mother? Who is my real father? Who is the authentic mother? Who is the authentic father? Must a real mother be genetically related? Does a man have the right to detach himself without responsibility from his sperm? And, not least of all, the question with which adoptees are still struggling: Is genetic relatedness necessary for an authentic sense of self?

Of course, the scenario of our brave new baby will have unique questions. What if he learns that his mother's egg and his father's sperm met in a saucer and he shacked up in a stranger's womb? Would the woman in whose womb he was implanted, on whose body fluid he fattened, on whose umbilical cord he clung, but to whom he was not genetically related, be a stranger, or would she be his mother? What if the brave new baby learns that her father took money as an anonymous donor to a sperm bank or paid money to have his sperm impregnate an anonymous woman? Can a child endure having an anonymous father or an anonymous mother? Would that child feel anonymous or unborn, as many adoptees do?

What if he learns that he had a surrogate mother who carried him for a price in her womb and gave him up like a piece of merchandise after he was born? Could she be called a mother, or even human? Would she be seen as less than human — little more than a glass jar?

Surrogate mothers differ from birth mothers who surrender their children for adoption in that they make a calculated business deal from the beginning. The typical birth mother who gives her child for adoption is young, unmarried, and pressured by her family to give up the baby. Studies show that these women often suffer from depression for the rest of their lives. Concerned United Birth Parents, a national group organized in the last decade, has been fighting to dispel the societal myth that all birth parents want privacy, in fact, many want the legal right to know what happened to their children. Adoptees are usually able to forgive their birth mothers when they learn the true story behind their relinquishment. But the question is—can our brave new baby ever forgive a surrogate mother?

Unless all surrogate mothers prove to be like Marybeth Whitehead who, as of this writing, is still in court fighting to keep her baby—known nationally as Baby M—our brave new surrogate babies are going to have a lot of feelings of rage, and a sense of worthlessness. Whatever the judge decides is in the best interest of Baby M—to stay with her father, William Stern, and to be adopted by his wife, or to return to her mother, Mary Beth Whitehead and her husband, Baby M's best interest will not be served. As in adoption cases, she will be cut off from one half of her heritage unless a custody arrangement is worked out in which she has the right to know both her biological mother and her biological father while she is growing up. If Marybeth Whitehead's legal rights are terminated, as birth mothers' are in adoption cases, then Baby M will be the loser—as are all adoptees in the present closed adoption system—in that she will not be able to integrate the truth of her heritage while she is growing up. Like many adoptees, she may act out her anger and grief in her adolescence or young adulthood.

In spite of the perils inherent in surrogate contracts, as illustrated by the Baby M case, most states are already working on legislation that would safeguard such arrangements by having the mothers' rights legally terminated before the birth of the baby. Better interview techniques have been suggested to insure that only those women who can easily give up a child be selected. But what kind of woman can easily give up a child? And what kind of society wants to encourage this kind of woman?

The questions are endless: we will need a new vocabulary to answer them. In the adoption world there is already a vocabulary war. Adoptive parents insist upon calling the mothers who gave birth to the child the biological mother rather than the natural mother, because the latter would imply that adoptive mothers were unnatural. The natural mothers insist that they be called the birth mother because the term biological does not sound human or caring. Surely the reproductive technology revolution will produce, along with babies, new terminology to battle over: the sperm donor, the genetic parent, the gestation parent, the surrogate uterus, the surrogate mother, the psychological mother and the genetic mother.

Whatever combinations and definitions we make, I hope we will at least relinquish the secrecy that has been the scourge of the adoption system, that we will be open and honest with this brave new baby. And however our baby started out in this world — frozen, fertilized, implanted, or transplanted — I hope he or she will grow up to be a writer or artist who can depict for us not only what it is like in the wine dark sea of a rented womb, but what the world looks like through the crystalline clarity of a glass test tube.

REFERENCES

Lifton, B. J. 1979. *Lost and Found, The Adoption Experience*. New York: Dial Press. 1988. Harper & Row.

Lifton, B. J. *Twice Born, Memoirs of an Adopted Daughter*. New York: Penguin: 1977.

C. L. Gaylord. 1976. "The Adoptive Child's Right To Know." *Case and Comment*.

J. Triseliotis. 1973. *In Search of Origins; The Experiences of Adopted People*. London: Routledge and Kegan Paul.

Arthur D. Sorosky, Annette Baran, and Reuben Pannor. 1978. *The Adoption Triangle: The Effects of the Sealed Record on Adoptees, Birth Parents and Adoptive Parents*. New York: Anchor Press/Doubleday.

The Changing Face of Adoption. 1977. (Report of Research Project, Children's Home Society of California.)

Norman Paul. 1973. "On a Child's Need for a Sense of Intergenerational Continuity: The Need to Know One's Roots." (Paper prepared for the G.A.P. Committee on the Family.)

Phyllis R. Silverman. 1981. *Helping Women Cope With Grief*. Beverly Hills, London: Sage Publications.

In Vitro Fertilization: Ethical Issues

Thomas A. Shannon

SUMMARY. This paper presents an overview of ethical issues concerning IVF. The first section evaluates specific ethical issues; the medical understanding of IVF, the development of the procedure, the risks of the procedure, and issues related to consent. The second part of the paper reviews broader issues: the allocation of resources, who receives the benefits, implications of IVF, and feminist issues. This review of ethical issues presents a framework to understand and evaluate the value dimensions raised by this technology.

In 1978, I wrote my first article on *in vitro* fertilization (IVF). This article commented on the birth of Louise Brown, the first human born of IVF, and was critical of the enterprise (Shannon 1978). In that article. I critiqued the process in light of the following issues: (1) the problem of the allocation of resources: (2) the ethics of experimentation including the possibility of coerced consent and the problem of the unconsenting subject of such research: (3) concerns about the irresolution of infertility: (4) the impact of competition in science. Here I wish to amplify some of those early concerns and raise other issues about the technology of IVF. My comments will focus on two areas: ethical issues specific to the technology of IVF itself and broader social issues.

I. ETHICAL ISSUES SPECIFIC TO THE TECHNOLOGY OF IVF

A. Medical

If the purpose of medicine is to restore a person to health, in what respect is someone who is infertile unhealthy? Surely the desires, hopes, and plans of that individual may be dashed and they may suffer as a consequence of their infertility, but are they unhealthy? In all respects but this one, they are biologically functional and healthy.

Is infertility a disease? That is, how do we categorize infertility so that we can understand its place in the discipline of medicine? Clearly, infertility is a consequence of some malfunction in the reproductive system which results in the inability of a couple to have a child (Kass 1985: 157ff). If having a child is a biological necessity, then classifying infertility as a disease is more understandable. But if having a child is a desire, a "want" instead of a "need," then infertility, while still serious, may be less easily understood as a disease.

Understood as a biological malfunction, infertility is a disease. Even so, infertility is a strange disease. Its presence may show up only as a consequence of not being able to conceive: other than that, individuals may not know they are infertile. They become aware of the malfunction only when they seek to exercise a choice. Other than in that one instance — and obviously the consequences that flow from it — their lives are unaffected by it.

Unless one is consciously seeking to have a child, one can essentially remain unaffected by the disease of infertility all of one's life. For example, many individuals who take vows of celibacy or choose not to have children, or remain single may be in fact infertile, but their lives are not affected by their infertility in any meaningful way.

The next question, then, is, "How does IVF affect infertility?" The answer is that IVF does not affect infertility, it only resolves childlessness. If the individuals were infertile before IVF, they are just as infertile afterwards. In some respects, the relief of symptoms is typical of what medicine frequently does. Insulin does not cure diabetes, contact lenses do not cure myopia, nor does Intal cure asthma. But all of these interventions certainly make life more bearable and increase the quality of life. Thus the couple needs to understand that IVF does not resolve infertility and consider whether symptomatic relief is sufficient for them.

As helpful as these interventions are, they are compensations, rather than cures. Even the best extended wear contact lenses are still contact lenses and the individual can't see well without them. And if infertility is the cause of individuals' distress and depression, then those feelings of inferiority or inadequacy may yet remain after successful IVF therapy. Perhaps such feelings may be increased because the individual knows that the only way of having a biological child is through a very complex technical process.

Thus infertility remains in a strange place. Though an abnormality and a malfunction of the reproductive system, if it is a disease, it is an unusual disease. It effects very little of an individual's physiology and becomes an issue only when conception is discovered to be impossible. Unlike selective abortion for genetic indications which cures the disease by eliminating the patient, IVF eliminates the symptoms by creating new individuals.

A closely related issue is "What is the function of medicine?" Should medicine be used to cure disease or to respond to the desires of individuals and the values of the culture? It is one thing to respond to the desires of an aging male to have his youthful appearance restored through surgical means, and quite another to develop the process of IVF to resolve childlessness. But the recipient of either procedure may not be any healthier after the medical intervention than before.

Thus IVF raises serious concerns about the nature of disease and medicine and how they relate to our desires and hopes. The fact that scientists, physicians, and technical procedures are involved does not necessarily mean that infertility is a disease or that the infertile person is unhealthy. Such individuals and their technologies may ensure that a problem is solved. But the problem that is solved may not be the one that is the real source of concerns.

B. The Development of the Procedure

The main concern here is whether or not there has been too fast an application of IVF to humans. The first confirmed external fertilization of a mammal egg occurred in 1959 when Dr. Chang of the Worcester Foundation for Experimental Biology fertilized a rabbit egg. By 1971, Drs. Steptoe and Edwards had perfected the technique of the external fertilization of a human egg. And in 1978, a live birth resulted from such an externally fertilized egg.

A nineteen-year span from the successful external fertilization of a rabbit egg to the live birth of a human conceived externally may not seem an unacceptably short time. Additional animal work was done during that same time span. Thus IVF is not without biological precedents. Yet Steptoe and Edwards did not do that much animal work themselves, nor have many of the clinics now in existence begun by establishing animal models.

We seem to have moved quite rapidly from some animal research to a full blown clinical application of the IVF procedure. And while this does not necessarily suggest that the professionals involved are irresponsible, some questions are necessarily raised. Has the procedure been researched as thoroughly as necessary? Who sets the standards for safety and how are they set? Should there be regulation of the developing industry of artificial reproduction and who should set the regulations? We have moved quickly from modest research to clinical application.

Thus far, the published record of human IVF has been encouraging with respect to the safety of the egg and the woman. Yet there is a continued need for a thorough study of the safety of the procedure, the biological development of the fertilized egg, the impact of hormones used to stimulate ovulation and the safety of the implantation procedure.

C. Risks of the Procedure

The primary risks for the woman are associated with the procedure of harvesting the egg(s) (Corea 1985: 173ff). To ensure a sufficient number of eggs, hormonal treatment is initiated. This causes several eggs to mature so an ample supply will be ensured in case the first fertilization and implantation efforts fail. As yet, no detrimental effects have been associated with this use of hormones. However, careful monitoring is required to determine whether or not there might be any long term consequences. Additionally, the aspiration procedures for obtaining the eggs can harm the ovary itself. The laparoscopy needed to obtain the egg exposes the woman to the risk of general anesthesia and possible infection from the surgery itself.

Once the egg has been fertilized, it needs to be placed within the uterus. This procedure exposes the woman to two additional risks: the possibility of the perforation of the uterus by the catheter during the implantation procedure and the possibility of infection of the uterus resulting from the procedure.

After the pregnancy is established, a number of monitoring procedures are typically used. These include ultrasound, amniocentesis, and endometrial biopsy. These are standard practice for many pregnancies and some safety evaluations have been made on them, especially amniocentesis. Ultrasound monitoring is a relatively new procedure and, although it is apparently risk free or at least low risk, studies should be initiated to determine that it is risk free.

Finally, there is the risk of an ectopic pregnancy resulting from the misplacement of the fertilized egg. This presents the most severe threat to the woman's health. While not a frequent occurrence, an ectopic pregnancy is a real possibility and monitoring for this situation is required.

Harm to the egg can occur at four points in the IVF procedure. First, the egg is at risk during the process of forced maturity because hormone therapy is used to induce superovulation. Second, the egg is at risk during the retrieval process. Third, the egg can be harmed while being manipulated during the process of fertilization and reimplantation. Fourth, the fertilized egg is at risk from the monitoring procedures to which it is subjected.

D. Clinical Studies

To determine what is happening in the field of artificial reproduction, one has to read a great number of both scientific and popular journals. There is no national registry to which data are reported, and essentially anyone with a medical degree can open a reproduction clinic without having to meet any standards. Thus it is very difficult to know what is actually happening. Some studies summarize the limited data available, but there is a genuine need to establish a national registry of research and practice in the reproductive technologies (Grobstein et al. 1983: 123).

Agreement also needs to be reached on how to determine and report success rates. Does one report, for example, the numbers of pregnancies obtained, the pregnancies per laparoscopy, the pregnancies per embryo transfer, the live births per pregnancy, the live births per laparoscopy, or the live births per transfer? Obviously the method of reporting makes a huge difference in what the success rate appears to be. Consistency is called for here.

Finally the practice of IVF is unregulated by federal, state, or professional standards (Andrews 1985: American Fertility Society, 1986). To "open shop," one simply needs to be a physician. This is potentially dangerous for the consumer. The physician may not necessarily be an obstetrician, may report the data one way to suggest higher success rate, and may not have the appropriate equipment or facilities to decrease the risks to the woman. The desperation of infertile couples and the unregulated nature of the practice of IVF may create too high a potential for serious conflicts of interests. Professional medical societies are now establishing standards which will help resolve some of these problems.

E. Informed Consent

The process of obtaining consent to a medical procedure is always difficult. People hear what they want to and ignore what is difficult or painful. Additionally, some relevant and important clinical information is difficult for a layperson to comprehend. Obtaining consent for the process of IVF has specific difficulties.

The population seeking IVF is a vulnerable one. The individuals have exhausted all other methods of having children biologically related to them and turn to this as their last resort. They may be desperate, driven people for whom no risk may be too great. Such a psychological condition may decrease their appreciation of the information they are given, may lead them to inappropriately discount the risks associated with the procedure, and may cause them to misunderstand or ignore the success rate of a particular clinic.

The vulnerability of this population of infertile couples leaves them open to misunderstanding of information correctly and appropriately provided, self-deception induced by their own desires, and manipulation by the unscrupulous practitioner. Particular care needs to be taken with these individuals so that they understand the risks and benefits of IVF.

II. BROADER ETHICAL ISSUES

A. The Allocation of Resources

One of the critical issues that IVF raises is the problem of how medical procedures and costs ought to be allocated. IVF obviously requires money, staff, and equipment. If large amounts of resources are used for artificial reproduction, obviously those same resources cannot be used elsewhere.

In 1983, the ". . . aggregate costs [were] about $50,000 . . ." for each child born from IVF procedures (Grobstein et al., 1983: 130). While the potential population for IVF varies with the particular fertility problem(s) of the individual, Grobstein estimates that if insurance were available, about 35,000 individuals could seek IVF annually (Grobstein et al. 1983: 130). That turns out to be a cost of $1.75 billion each year to produce IVF babies. And that is without calculating the costs of malpractice insurance, staff costs, and overhead.

Where should these funds come from? Insurance premiums would have to rise dramatically to cover these costs. And given the current level of the federal deficits, there will probably not be much enthusiasm for federal funding.

Additionally the funding issue will force more directly the question of whether the procedure is genuinely therapeutic or is treating individuals' wishes. The public funding argument may be more successful if the procedure is determined to be genuinely therapeutic. But one still needs to determine where infertility treatment fits in the hierarchy of other health issues.

B. For Whose Benefit?

Closely related to the funding issue is the issue of who benefits from the procedure. The impression one receives from the literature is that most IVF clients are white and upper or upper middle class. Few minorities have the resources of time and money to travel to a clinic and stay there for several weeks until conception occurs.

Can the estimated $1.75 billion be a justified expenditure when it benefits such a narrow band of the population? Will one hear resurrected concerns about the poor overpopulating themselves and needing increased welfare benefits as the basis for denying IVF to the poor? If IVF is publicly funded, it must be open to everyone.

Clearly the scientists at work on IVF and similar technologies are motivated by the desire to help individuals who are suffering. They also want to increase knowledge. The possibility of understanding the totality of the reproductive process, as well as the capacity to control it is a powerful motivator. The desire to be first with a process or procedure is also strong. Many breakthroughs are yet to come in the areas of artificial reproduction, and fame and fortune await the discoverers. Competition is a powerful motivator in science.

This mixed motivation in the clinician-scientist has the potential to confuse priorities by putting knowledge for knowledge's sake, or a prize, ahead of the patient. Whether this happens can only be determined on a case by case basis. Nonetheless the conflict of interest is present and, given the history of research, such conflicts can have serious consequences.

C. Implications of IVF

The most significant feature of IVF, in my judgement, is that the process of conception is external and renders the fertilized egg accessible to manipulation.

Who controls what is done to the fertilized egg? Presumably as long as the parents are alive, they are the ones to determine that. But, typically, several eggs are fertilized to serve as back-ups in case the first implant doesn't work. Should the couple from whom the sperm and egg were obtained retain control over these "extra" fertilized eggs if they are not needed? When the egg or sperm come from a third party, who retains control then?

Frequently extra fertilized eggs are not destroyed, but are frozen to serve as a back-up, or to avoid the need for another laparoscopy if another pregnancy is desired. What is the moral status of the blastocyst while it is frozen? What is the moral status of the blastocyst while it is frozen? Who maintains control of it and for how long? The case of the frozen "orphan embryos" in Australia several years ago illustrates the nature of the dilemma. Many clinics now have formal or informal guidelines or policies on these issues, such as having the parents state their long term wishes for the disposition of the frozen blastocyst. But such policies are idiosyncratic to the particular clinic and may have no legal standing.

Such policies also put the blastocyst into a new social role: patient. And although the blastocyst may have no civil rights, the blastocyst-as-patient may have some rights with respect to medical care, nondiscriminatory treatment, and maintenance of life support system. Minimally the social role of blastocyst-as-patient will confuse even further how we understand that entity. At the most, we may seriously need to reconsider whether the blastocyst has civil and moral rights.

Finally, since the fertilized egg is accessible, it is subject to the possibility of genetic engineering. We are in the beginning stages of gene therapy, and having research material in various stages of embryonic development may be a boon for its development. Of course, once one learns how to intervene therapeutically in the gene, then the door is open to other types of modifications. Many of the elements to begin a program of genetic engineering are in place.

D. Feminist Issues

Of the many issues that artificial reproduction raises for women, two in particular stand out. First, most IVF clinics require heterosexual marriage as a prerequisite for enrollment in the program. Presumably, the primary motivation for this requirement is to gain social acceptability for the programs. But this requirement also denies children to others and raises the issue of whether or not one has a right to have children. And, granted such a right, it is coupled with the complementary question of whether a private program or one not subsidized by federal funds must service anyone who applies.

Second, is IVF yet another expression of the pronatalist bias in our culture? (Blake 1974: 159ff). This bias assumes that the question is *when* one will have children, not *whether* one will have them. This bias contributes, first, to the continued disenfranchisement of childless couples in our society. Second, it reinforces the assumption that one is not fully an adult until one has a child. Thus a childless woman is doubly disenfranchised.

Such a bias, and the technologies that express it, also reinforce the perspective that the primary or exclusive role of women is to have children. An assumption may be that a female is not fully a woman until she has been able to bear a child. There is an implicit affirmation that the worth of a woman is centered on her ability to reproduce. This attitude reinforces stereotypes of women and helps keep them in their subordinate social position. It reinforces attitudes that claim women's worth is derived from biology, not ability.

Thus the technology of IVF implicitly supports and contributes to many of our cultural stereotypes about women. Although IVF certainly helps some women achieve their dreams, it may keep many others from realizing theirs.

CONCLUSION

This essay has identified several ethical issues surrounding the development and use of IVF. Some of these issues are speculative and long term, which underscores the need to develop long-term monitoring. Other issues are immediate and suggest that present applications of IVF deserve scrutiny.

As a society we have handled IVF as we have other technologies. We have not asked the question of *whether* we should engage in IVF, but *how* we should do it. In traditional American fashion we have bypassed the most critical ethical questions and gone forward assuming that the risk-benefit issue is the only relevant question.

IVF is in place, it is accepted as part of the clinical treatment of infertility, and it is understood as another blessing of science and medicine. Yet few of the individuals who developed this technique questioned its impact on society or on women, its impact on already scarce medical resources, or its relation to other technologies such as genetic engineering. We have developed a technology that has profound consequences for the individual and, in typical American fashion, we assume that all will be right—or that any problems can be solved later.

Perhaps the social role of the ethicist is to be a professional worrier. Clearly other professions and individuals do not seem to be greatly concerned with the issues I have raised. Our American love affair with technology has been characterized by optimism, success, and a great deal of luck. Perhaps this story will be continued with IVF. Let us hope so, for we literally hold the conception of a new world in the palm of our hand.

REFERENCES

American Fertility Society. 1986. "Ethical Considerations of the New Reproductive Technologies." *Fertility and Sterility* 46 (September). This is a supplement to the September issue.

Andrews, L. B. 1984. *New Conceptions: A Consumer's Guide to the Newest Infertility Treatments*. New York: St. Martin's Press.

Blake, J. 1974. "Coercive Pronatalism and American Population Policy." In *Pronatalism, Mom, and Apple Pie*, by Ellen Peck and Judy Benderowitz. New York: Thomas Y. Crowell Co.

Corea, G. 1985. *The Mother Machine*. New York: Harper and Row.

Grobstein, C. et al. 1983. "External Human Fertilization: An Evaluation of Policy." *Science* 222 (14 October): 122-133.

Kass, L. 1985. *Toward A More Natural Science*. New York: The Free Press.

Shannon, T. A. 1978. "The Case Against Test Tube Babies." *The National Catholic Reporter*. 11 August: 20.

Moral Reflections
on the New Technologies:
A Catholic Analysis

Ronald D. Lawler

SUMMARY. New technologies of conception bring into being beautiful babies. The wonder of these children, and of the technologies themselves, can tempt us to abbreviate ethical reflection on the moral appropriateness of initiating human life in this way. However, the moralists of the Catholic Church, along with many others, judge that human life should originate in acts of love between parents, not in productive acts of technologists. Scientific help for people desiring to generate a child out of their own being should be distinguished from scientific substitution for human acts of love in originating life. The child must be recognized as an equal, not as a product, subject to quality control. To radically alter our ways of generating human life without sufficient moral reflection is to generate human pain and moral dilemmas that we have not begun to fathom.

"The last time I saw her," Dr. Robert Edwards said of the newly born Louise Brown, the first test-tube baby, "she was just eight cells in a test tube. She was beautiful then, and she's beautiful now" (in P. Gynne 1978:7). Artificial technologies of conception lead to good results: wonderful human beings, astonishing skill, and important knowledge.

Unfortunately, it is also true that the worst moments in medical morality can come when—precisely because we are in pursuit of important goals—we neglect adequate ethical reflection. It is especially easy to make major moral errors when questionable behavior seems to pay off so well; yet while we seem to have grand reasons for rushing forward, our actions may not honor sufficiently every human value.

In the nineteenth century, when new technologies of artificial generation were first experimentally applied to humans, the overwhelming majority of Catholic theologians judged that it was irresponsible and immoral to use such procedures. This has been the consistent judgment of the Catholic Church in this matter.[1] The Church insists that its position is not a mere policy decision, nor a precept based on arcane religious motives; rather it argues that this position is a necessary defense of essential human values. The Church considers it appropriate to require a rational justification of such a judgment and believes that the "natural law," which is accessible to all independent of any faith commitment, requires that such activity be excluded. As one would expect, there are many moralists, not guided by particularly religious motives who are led by the same respect for important human values, and who hold and defend the same positions.[2]

Efforts to assist parents to have a "child of their own" have taken many forms. The end is certainly a good one, and many means used to reach it are surely morally upright. Some of the methods are very simple: conception is sometimes achieved when spouses learn more precisely the times and circumstances in which their acts of sexual love are more likely to be fruitful. Other methods are far more complex, yet offer no special moral problems, for example, various kinds of microsurgery and other therapeutic techniques which overcome the obstacles that have kept couples from generating their own children in acts of spousal love. These approaches not only escape the moral objections and many of the bitterly painful personal and social consequences of such techniques as *in vitro* fertilization, the remedy they provide is also corrective, generally less burdensome, and has a success rate which in most cases is notably higher.[3]

But methods such as IVF replace the parental generative act by something more akin to the manufacturing of babies. Skilled technicians produce babies out of material drawn from the would-be parents and/or others. The new human life is created not from an act of human love, but in a spirit of craftsmanlike "making." We are on the brink of the "brave new world" (Huxley 1932) that many of us would not wish.

When a new human life comes to be out of an act of love between two persons who will forever be parents, and responsible to the child — a child not made but begotten, not a product that its makers may manipulate, but an offspring that is their equal — the entire context suggests an attitude and a moral stance different from that which arises when human life is originated in the context of production, manufacturing, and quality control.

The context of "product-making" is clearly revealed in the way that *in vitro* production of children has proceeded. In *in vitro* clinics, more embryos are produced than are needed. Each of these embryos is in fact a distinctive and irreplaceable instance of humanity and deserves awe from the start. When they are first created, we can see their preciousness — "Eight cells and already lovely!" in Dr. Edwards' words. But awe seems not to have a home in the productive atmosphere: in due time the embryos that meet our standards and needs are used and the rest are casually destroyed.

"Eight cells and already lovely!" It is obvious, that in a sense any human being can be described as a collection of cells. But it is not clear that every "set of human cells" is alike in worth. The cells taken from human skin or flesh, and kept alive for a while, are indeed human cells; but these cells are not all that Louise Brown was when she was only eight cells. In such a mere cluster of cells there is not a new individual human life. But in the eight cells that Louise once was, there was a dynamic unity, a new instance of an utterly distinctive human life. Already she bore within herself the dynamism that would lead her in an entirely continuous physiological and psychological development toward full maturity.

Obviously the question of abortion accompanies the practice of *in vitro* fertilization. Catholic moral thought, like many other forms of moral thought today, holds that wherever a distinctive new entity of humankind comes into being, this being has important rights. Under this doctrine, to be considered a "person," one need only be a distinct and individual human being: one need not also be of a certain age, or a certain race, or in a certain stage of development (and those who demand that "being a person" involves something more cannot specify just what else is needed). Every distinct individual of the human species, embryo or adult, has the full rights of a person.

Still, opposition to abortion is certainly not the key objection to the *in vitro* generation of children. In principle it would certainly be possible to engage in *in vitro* fertilization without disposing of the new human beings as though they were mere clusters of cells.

The objection to reproductive technologies is simpler and more universal: to generate children by technological acts which separate the origin of life from acts of interpersonal love is not a good way to act. Such technological making of babies is irresponsible and immoral whatever we expect to come of it. The moral thinking that for centuries has guided humankind (not only in the great Judeo-Christian tradition, but also in the traditions of the East, much of classical paganism, and in Enlightenment thought with its inherited convictions of inalienable rights) has held that there are some kinds of acts which a moral person will refuse ever to do, or at least refuse to do except in "abnormal, painful, and improbable circumstances."[4]

Thus moral thinking common to the world's great religious, philosophical, and literary traditions has led to convictions that we ought not do evil that good may come of it, and that a number of possible ways of acting are in fact wrong. Thus, for example, deliberately killing an innocent person is held to be wicked, not simply because we would then all be in danger of similar acts but because killing innocent people is simply the wrong sort of thing to do. There are parallel reasons why moralists who remain in any of the great historical moral traditions that guided the consciences of most people over the centuries reject technological modes or producing human life. They believe that acts of basic and fundamental importance in human life should not be separated from the values that give them meaning and dignity. Just as speech should not be separated from the value of truth (so that lying is a wrong kind of act), and as acts of sexual intimacy should not be separated from concern for the personal good of the partner (so that seduction is wrong), so the creation of human life should not be separated from acts of interpersonal love. It is wrong to bring new individual humans into being as things crafted or produced by technical skills. Reverence for human life demands that the creation of new life should never be separated from free interpersonal acts of human love.

These forms of moral thinking are not automatically transferred from one generation to the next (education in virtue has commonly been held to be at once the most difficult and the most important task of every culture). These forms of moral thinking often stand in conflict with our passions and individual interests. They often stand in conflict with modes of thinking which are valid and necessary for some elements of human thought and progress, but which are not serviceable in guarding human values that are always in need of defense.

The well-publicized split between diverse cultural groups and, in our era, between scientific cultures and humanistic cultures is hard to define. It is regrettable that ethical decisions have become extremely hard to discuss across cultural barriers with the seriousness they deserve — and this at a time when new, very complex problems of immense importance need profound and shared consideration. To scientists, it often seems that humanists concerned with "old" values utterly fail to see how profoundly modern discoveries have changed the world. To humanists, it often seems that those who have had too little leisure to reflect on the personal values at stake suffer from philosophical naiveté. This makes them confuse what might be demanded by modern science and modern circumstances with what is demanded by unreflective acceptance of ideological assumptions about what constitutes human progress. Two things seem evident: (1) it is extremely important that there be broad and profound moral reflection on the serious value questions involved in decisions that are too often pressured by an unreflective "technological imperative"; (2) recent attempts to provide "professional ethics" training for scientific professionals to help bridge the gap between cultures have often been very shallow and unsuccessful.[5]

The essential ethical question is: Should we utilize the new technologies of generating life because they are effective in meeting certain concrete human needs and desires in spite of the objections that arise out of many traditional and contemporary moral visions? It is an ethical question that can not be easily answered with the assistance of quick courses in moral logic or in rhetorical encounters in which one side argues past the other. The question is much deeper: it is a question of the meaning of human values, what it means to be a person, what love and sexuality are, and how (and if) they should be related to the originating of life.

Traditional morality is concerned with acknowledging the relatedness of values. In traditional Catholic morality, for example, questions of proper ways to initiate human life are inseparable from reflection on the meaning of human love and sexuality, on differences between summoning new life into being by acts of human love and by acts of artful making. In this moral vision, the act of sexual love itself is held to be one of great depth and meaning. Sexual activity should reflect the kind of love its human reality symbolizes: a free and generous mutual self-giving, a pledge of the kind of faithful and cooperative love that also serves to make those pledging such love more suited to be both sources of new life and more suitable to sustain and care for such life. Human life should be created only in an act of sexual love between those who in that act can become parents.

One may object, of course, that acts of sexual intercourse are not the only acts of personal love. It may be added that the whole enterprise of artificial conception is in the service of love. Couples so seek children through artificial means because of great love. And the reason why creative minds have shaped the new technologies is that they wish to help people have the babies they long for.

There is some truth in this; but I am not sure that it is entirely true. The whole business of manufacturing babies could be motivated entirely by love if we assume there are not motives of careerism, pursuit of power to control, and social pressures. But the manufacturing is not of its nature an act of love, as is the act of marital love that generates a child. Catholic morality teaches that acts of sexual love are acts of great dignity and importance; it does not share the view of many that there is something unseemly about sex, and that it really might be even better if we could separate the important business of originating children from sex and human love in its most intensely personal form.[6]

It has been objected that children are often generated in sexual acts that are far from being either acts of love or acts motivated by love. Children are often born, "as the products of unilateral sexual aggressiveness, sometimes aggressiveness to the point of brutality, even within the marital unit, particularly so in cultures where the will of the father is the law of the household."[7] It may be asked then: is a skillful reproductive intervention, offered to satisfy a couple's longing for children, really more dehumanizing than an unreciprocated act of passion, which may involve little love?

Certainly I would say that acts of sexual intercourse that are not acts of mutual love and self-giving, are not proper acts in which human lives should be generated. But a flourishing IVF industry will not lessen the number of such acts, nor will institutionalizing and encouraging the creation of humans by acts that are not acts of love (even if they are very sophisticated and intelligent acts) be a step forward for the human race. It is not good for us to separate the beginning of life from acts of profound human loving, either replacing them by technology, or deforming them by sexual acts that do not express love.

Questions about the morality of *in vitro* fertilization, about artificial insemination, or about the use of surrogate mothers, are often evaded by naive suppositions that sensible people are simply handling specific practical questions now, and that the moral probings of others are rooted in some sort of strange religiosity or some outmoded forms of thinking. "Here are people who want children of their own, who clearly have a right to such children, and whom we can assist in having children of their own. Please get out of our way!"

In fact, this no-nonsense approach to artificial generation is full of unanalyzed and highly questionable claims. What is meant by "children of their own"? Children born both of their parents' flesh and blood, and also out of acts of love? Or is it enough that children be born out of materials from parents' bodies? Or from the body of at least one of them? Or do they mean parents have rights to children because they have contracted for the use of other materials and methodologies and have rented other wombs? Or children produced entirely in glass or various types of surrogate wombs, and assigned to "suitable" parents by appropriate officials?

And what is meant by saying people "clearly" have a "right" to "children of their own" in one or more of the above senses? Is the right to have a "child of my own" such an absolute one that demands we alter radically one of the most profoundly emotional and value-laden areas of our life, even before we have time to think clearly and come to a reasonable moral consensus? Is it right for us to encourage an atmosphere in which obvious and subtle pressures create an abortion industry that destroys a million and a half unborn babies every year, and then begin to establish another industry to create babies for people who are induced to believe that the baby someone manufactures for them will be more appropriate than a baby already living?

We are only beginning to see how immense are the moral problems that accompany artificially generated life. Everyone knows of the case (in Australia) of two embryos brought into being by IVF techniques from genetic materials of a wealthy Australian couple (actually the sperm was from another man.) The would-be parents died in a plane accident, while the embryos were in a frozen state awaiting possible implantation. The embryos became a focus of national attention: should they be allowed to develop to maturity, and perhaps become millionaires? or should they simply be disposed of? It is not an isolated question, when we begin new human lives as products of our technology, and not as offspring generated by acts of love.

The Whitehead-Stern surrogate mother case in New Jersey also illustrates the dilemmas created when decisions touching the central roots of human life, love, and conviction are made too hastily. When babies are brought into being in such a way, it is not possible to take into account intelligently the profound claims of the various persons involved. The "technological imperative" is a cruel one — we can do this wonderful thing of "making your own baby for you," so we feel we must do it — when it does not take into account more sophisticated moral thinking than the hasty belief that "if something does some good for somebody, it is reasonable to do it." When we fix our eyes only on the good effects hoped for, we forget the pain created too; we forget that artificial forms of generation remain very expensive, accessible to few; that they take resources that are desperately needed elsewhere; that *in vitro* fertilization works for relatively few people, and that failure to succeed even after such heroic efforts is so psychologically painful. We forget that other ways of bringing the joy of children into people's lives have far greater success rates, without any special moral problems, and without any implications of "brave new world."

The longing of people to have children is real, and the concern of scientists to help is praiseworthy. But morality is largely a matter of means. And we have a duty to reflect more seriously on the morality of our new technological means of generating human life, before intolerable harm is done to too many people's lives.

NOTES

1. See the recent document published by the Congregation for the Doctrine of the Faith, Instruction on Respect for Human Life in its Origin and on the Dignity of Procreation (Vatican City, 1987). The first firm teaching of the Church on the subject is found in a Decree of the Holy Office of March 17, 1887, insisting flatly that artificial insemination of women is illicit (Denzinger n. 3323). Important subsequent elucidations of this are found in documents of Pope Pius XII in 1949 and 1951 (Denzinger n. 3954). An article in the *New Catholic Encyclopedia* (McKeever 1967) reveals how universal Catholic acceptance of this position was; only in very recent years has there been some retreat from it by some. For a survey of Catholic teaching on the subject, see the 1984 article of Fitzgerald noted in the bibliography.

2. In fact, in recent years leadership in defense of the traditional view that human persons should be generated only in acts of human love has been given chiefly by scholars of Protestant and secular background, such as Paul Ramsey and Leon Kass (Ramsey 1970, 1972; Kass 1971, 1972), although important work continues to be done by Catholic scholars (Santamaria 1984; May 1983).

3. For an argument that microsurgery approaches should be used in most of the cases in which at present *in vitro* fertilization is often used, see the 1984 article of Dr. Peter Peterson, given at a conference on the subject in Melbourne. Note for comparison that articles on parallel subjects (given at the same conference, and noted in the bibliography below) by Dr. Carl Wood and Dr. Robin Rowland.

4. Basil Mitchell (1980:137) points out how well-grounded are the reflective moral judgments that exclude on non-utilitarian grounds some kinds of acts that are offensive to human values and personal dignity. In a popular and well-known study, C.S. Lewis (1943) points out how broad and how strong is the support of the general moral position he chooses to call "*Tao*" with it vigorous insistence that some kinds of acts are not simply in fact widely disapproved, but objectively

and surely deserve to be repudiated, as really becoming for human persons to do. A more sophisticated defense of such values is found in Alasdair MacIntyre (1981).

5. Henry Veatch, an articulate defender of the classical natural law tradition, points out the immense flaws in most contemporary approaches to professional ethics in a special volume of *Listening* (1982), in which he gathers essays on the subject from a number of points of view.

6. This traditional Catholic position is forcefully stated in 1965 in the Second Vatican Council's *Pastoral Constitution on the Church in the Modern World*, n. 47-52. For further development of this theme, see Lawler (1985).

BIBLIOGRAPHY

Denzinger, H. and A. Schoenmetzer, eds. 1967. *Enchiridion Symbolorum*. Rome: Herder.

Fitzgerald, L. 1984. "IVF and Catholic Moral Teaching." In Santamaria, J. and N. Toni-Filippini, eds.:127-133.

Gynne, P. 1978. "Was the Birth of Louise Brown Only a Happy Accident?" *Science Digest* (Oct. 1978):7-12.

Huxley, A. 1932. *Brave New World*. New York and London: Harper and Row.

Kass, L. 1971. "Babies by Means of *In Vitro* Fertilization." *New England Journal of Medicine* 285 (1971):1174-1179.

Kass, L. 1972. "Making Babies: The New Biology and the "Old Morality." *The Public Interest* 26 (Winter 1972):28-56.

Lawler, R., J. Boyle, and W. May, 1985. *Catholic Sexual Ethics*. Huntington, Ind: OSV Press.

Lewis, C. S. 1943. *The Abolition of Man*. Oxford: University Press.

Mac Intrye, A. 1981. *After Virtue*. Notre Dame, Ind.: Univ. of Notre Dame Press.

Mc Keever, P. 1967. "Artificial Insemination." *New Catholic Encyclopedia*. Vol. 1. New York: McGraw Hill: 922-24.

May, W. 1983. "Begotten Not Made: Reflections on Laboratory Production of Human Life." In F. Lescoe, ed., *Perspectives in Bioethics*. New Britain, CT.: Mariel: 29-60.

Mitchell, B. 1980. *Morality: Religious and Secular*. Oxford: Clarendon Press.

Peterson, P. 1984. "Microsurgery." In J. Santamaria and N. Tonti-Filippin (1984): 117-125.

Ramsey, P. 1970. *Fabricated man*. New Haven: Yale University Press.

Ramsey, P. 1972. "Shall We Reproduce: I. The Medical Ethics of *In Vitro* Fertilization." *Journal of the American Medical Association* 220 (1972):1346-1350.

Rowland, R. "Social and Psychological Aspects." (1984). Proceedings of the *1984 Conference on Bioethics*. Melbourne: St. Vincent's Bioethic Centre.

Santamaria, J. and N. Tonti-Filippini, eds. 1984. *Proceedings of the 1984 Conference on Bioethics*. Melbourne: St. Vincent's Bioethic Centre.

Second Vatican Council. 1965. *Pastoral Constitution on the Church in the Modern World*.

Veatch, Henry. 1982. "Ethics and Applied Ethics: an Introductory Note." *Listening* 17 (Winter 1982):2-10.

Wood, C. 1984. "*In Vitro* Fertilization—The Procedure and Future Development." In J. Santamaria and N. Tonti-Filippini (1984):95-102.

Procreative Liberty, Embryos, and Collaborative Reproduction: A Legal Perspective

John A. Robertson

SUMMARY. This article discusses the implications of a constitutionally protected right to procreate using a wide range of reproductive choices made possible by noncoital reproductive technologies, including embryo freezing and donation and surrogate gestation. After establishing the constitutional basis for a positive right to procreate, it discusses the extent to which concerns about the welfare of embryos, offspring, donors, and surrogates justifies limitation on reproductive choice involving these technologies. While tangible harm to offspring and protection of the free choice of reproductive collaborators may justify regulation, moral condemnation of noncoital techniques and concerns about the reifying effects of their use are an insufficient basis for state restriction.

Procreative liberty has in recent years been most often discussed in terms of the negative right to avoid procreation through access to abortion and contraception. I want to discuss the "positive" aspect of procreative liberty—the liberty to procreate how and when one chooses—as it arises with technologically-assisted reproduction.

The positive right to procreate has not yet been extensively examined. The growing use of noncoital reproductive techniques now forces us to consider this aspect of procreative liberty. Developments in external fertilization and embryo transfer and the use of

This paper is an edited transcript of a talk given at York College, C.U.N.Y., in November, 1985. A longer version of it appears as "Embryos, Families and Procreative Liberty: the Legal Structure of the New Reproduction," 59 *Southern California Law Review* 501-601 (1986).

donors and surrogates require attention to such questions as: is there a right to reproduce noncoitally? Is there a right to reproduce non-coitally with the assistance of third party collaborators? What limits on noncoital reproduction are within state or professional power? Do notions of reproductive responsibility justify limitation of non-coital reproduction?

I will briefly discuss the constitutional status of the positive right to procreate, and then examine how embryo status, concerns for offspring and family, and more general concerns with the reifica-tion of reproduction influence the scope of individual use of the new reproductive technologies.

THE CONSTITUTIONAL STATUS OF A RIGHT TO PROCREATE

It is reasonable to conclude that married couples in the United States have a constitutionally protected right to reproduce by sexual intercourse. No laws have ever restricted marital reproduction and few court cases even discuss the issue. The state has never tried to interfere with the right of married couples to reproduce by coitus.

Two points that have great significance for the new reproductive technologies follow from constitutional acceptance of a married couple's right to reproduce coitally. First is the right of the married couple to reproduce noncoitally as well, through such means as artificial insemination with the husband's sperm or through extra-corporeal fertilization—the IVF process. Second, is the right to re-produce noncoitally with the assistance of donors and surrogates. If one or both partners lack the genetic or gestational elements neces-sary to procreate, it should follow that they have the right to enlist the willing assistance of donors and surrogates to provide the gam-etes or missing gestational function. Careful attention to the prece-dents, values, and interests that support protecting coital conception should lead to similar protection for noncoital reproduction.

If this analysis is correct, couples would have a constitutional right (e.g., a right against state interference with or prohibition of their actions) to create, store, transfer, donate and possibly even manipulate extra-corporeal embryos in order to acquire offspring of their genes or gestation for the purpose of rearing as their child.

Contracts with gamete and embryo donors and surrogates would also be constitutionally protected. Only very important state interests, such as tangible harm to other persons, would justify restricting noncoital and collaborative reproductive variations. Moral distaste alone would not be a sufficient ground for limiting procreative liberty, even though moral distaste might legitimately animate the private-sector decisions of patients and physicians.

The implication of this analysis for collaborative reproductive transactions needs special emphasis. It suggests that the contract among the parties concerning rearing rights and duties in offspring is presumptively controlling. Giving legal effect to the agreement that couples make with third-party collaborators limits state intervention to regulating the conditions of entering into such contracts, and leaves little room for restricting the substantive bargains struck among the parties. However, some restrictions to protect offspring may also be within the state's power.

I have emphasized the right of married couples because their right to reproduce is so firmly established in American law. One can make a very strong argument for unmarried persons, either single or as couples, also having a positive right to reproduce. This has not yet been explicitly recognized in American law. However, if their right to coital conception is recognized, then single and unmarried persons should have the same rights that married couples have to reproduce noncoitally and with the assistance of donors and surrogates.

This analysis of procreative rights answers many, but not all of the legal questions that arise concerning use of the new reproductive technology. The constitutional structure provides a framework that accords high value to procreative choice, but answers to specific disputes and problems may ultimately depend on the meanings people find in the reproductive roles that noncoital technology makes possible. One set of questions arises about the scope of partial reproductive roles. A woman now can be an egg donor and not a gestator just as a man may be a sperm donor. A woman may also choose to be a surrogate gestator to experience gestation without having a genetic tie with the offspring. What limits, if any, should be placed on women and men playing such partial reproductive roles?

Another set of questions concerns the right to reproduce posthumously through postmortem thawing of cryopreserved eggs, sperm, and embryos. Do these partial reproductive roles deserve the same respect and protection as reproductive roles that aim at producing offspring to be reared? Answers to these questions will depend on the meanings that people find in such experiences, and their relation to the interests and values that underlie the positive right to procreate.

EMBRYO STATUS

Let me turn now to various interests that have been put forward as grounds for limiting the positive right to procreate. One set of interests concern pre-implantation embryos. Concern for embryos has led some persons to support restrictions on what might be done with embryos. Such proposals require us to assess the legal and moral status of the extra-corporeal embryo. Does the pre-implantation embryo at any of its stages from fertilization, through zygote and blastocyst have legal or moral rights that limit what the gamete sources (biological parents) or others might do with it? What is the nature and moral status of this living, embryonic entity? We must address these questions to resolve the locus and limits of authority over preimplantation embryos.

Given the biological status of pre-implantation embryos, I have difficulty viewing the pre-implantation embryo as a rights-bearing entity by virtue of its existing characteristics. Whatever one thinks of the fetus at a later stage of development, the one or two or four or eight-celled embryo is not an entity that possesses rights by virtue of its present characteristics. The pre-implantation embryo lacks even the rudiments of a nervous system. It is not sentient, and is no more conscious than any other group of cells. Some religious and right-to-life groups view the pre-implantation embryo as a "person," but I think this view is mistaken, at least if we regard "person" as a being that is capable of cognition and consciousness and interaction. The embryo lacks even the most rudimentary characteristics that a person or any rights-bearing entity would have.

However, the embryo might still be accorded value as a symbol of human life generally. I want to make a distinction between owing the embryo respect by virtue of its existing characteristics, and according respect because of what it might become. While the embryo in itself may not yet be a rights-bearing entity, it clearly has the potential to attain the characteristics of persons, if certain contingencies occur. Persons may choose to invest the embryo with meaning as a symbol of human life generally, even though justice does not require that we protect it in any particular way. Particular efforts to demonstrate respect for the embryo as symbol, however, must meet constitutional standards.

If this analysis is correct, then the validity of limits on embryo manipulations depends on whether the embryo is going to be transferred to a uterus and thus has a possibility of implanting, going to term, and becoming a child. In that case embryos have a special legal and moral status, not in and of themselves by virtue of their present characteristics, but because of what they may become. Activities with embryos that may be transferred to a uterus could directly affect resulting offspring. There is a body of law relevant here that recognizes prenatal obligations to offspring and permits sanctions to be imposed on persons who knowingly or recklessly harm born children by prenatal actions. This same body of law would impose restrictions on embryo manipulations that could foreseeably harm children born after transfer of such embryos to a uterus.

Where transfer to a uterus is not planned or desired, the question of embryo status per se in my view is symbolic, rather than a matter of rights. What legal and moral status does the embryo have if it is not going to be transferred? This question is of importance with regard to the permissibility of research with nontransferred embryos, and the permissibility of destroying or not transferring embryos that are unwanted by the woman who contributed the egg. Because of space constraints, I will discuss only the question of not transferring unwanted embryos to a uterus.

Is there a moral or legal duty to transfer all embryos to a uterus so that they might have the chance to implant and come to term? At present there is no such legal duty, and few commentators who do not view the fertilized egg itself as a rights bearing human subject find a moral duty to do so. I would argue that nothing is owed the preimplantation embryo in itself. It is too rudimentary to be the object of justice in its own right. Persons may, nonetheless, choose to invest the embryo with value as a symbol of human life generally, even though they recognize that there is no moral obligation to do so.

The current practice in most of the 120 American IVF programs is to transfer all embryos to a woman's uterus. Although not legally required, this practice has developed for various reasons, including a desire to avoid controversy with right-to-life groups over abortion. Yet this practice now poses potential conflicts with the wishes of the couples providing the egg and sperm. The standard IVF regimen stimulates the production of multiple eggs. If more than four eggs are retrieved and fertilized, placement of all of them in the uterus produces a high risk of multiple gestation. To avoid this risk, it might be necessary to discard some of the embryos. Cryopreservation may postpone the decision, but eventually the question will arise, since transfer of these stored embryos at a later time may not be possible.

Persons who believe that the embryo itself has rights or that a symbolic statement about respect for human life should be made might support mandatory embryo donation laws. Such a law might read: "All extra-corporeal embryos that the woman who provided the egg does not want to have transfered to her must be transferred, with the donors anonymity guaranteed and no rearing duties imposed, to a willing recipient." Would a mandatory embryo donation law be constitutionally acceptable? Such a law does not violate a woman's right to have an abortion because it does not require that a woman accept placement of an embryo in her uterus. It would, however, lead to offspring unwanted by the biologic parents. Yet if no rearing rights and duties attach, and the donation is anonymous, the interest in avoiding unwanted biologic offspring might not be accorded constitutional protection.

Resolution of this conflict turns on our valuation of an unwanted biologic link. Is that a matter of great personal significance to individuals, so that a genetic link should not be created unless they consent? Or is that a minor concern that does not merit public protection when it is anonymous and imposes no undesired rearing rights and duties?

The answer to this question will evolve with the different uses to which reproductive technology is put. Ultimately the Supreme Court may have to decide the matter. In my view, the most desirable practice is to transfer all embryos where reasonably possible as a way of demonstrating respect for life generally. However, if people who have produced the genes for the embryo object, I think it probably best to leave the final decision with them. The symbolic gain from embryo sustaining is outweighed by the sources' wish to avoid an unwanted genetic connection. However, constitutionally, the state may be found to have authority to require donation of unwanted embryos, when rearing duties are not imposed on the genetic parents.

This discussion of embryo status reminds us not to assume that our views about abortion automatically indicate answers in the significantly different area of IVF and extra-corporeal embryos. The embryo differs from the fetus in two significant ways. The embryo is substantially less developed than a fetus, without organs, a brain or the most rudimentary cellular units of the neuromuscular system. One could logically be against abortion on the grounds of respect for the sentience of late-term fetuses, and at the same time hold that pre-implantation embryos may be discarded by the gamete source.

The second point of difference is that the extra-corporeal embryo, unlike the fetus, is not inside a woman, is not making demands on a woman's body. Therefore, one could be in favor of abortion, of allowing the woman to expel the fetus, and still permit state intervention to protect extra-corporeal embryos by requiring their donation to willing recipients because of the symbolic importance of demonstrating respect for human life in this way. Mandatory embryo donation does not impose physical burdens on a woman as anti-abortion laws would, and thus needs to be analyzed in terms of the impact of an unwanted genetic link.

FAMILY AND REARING ISSUES

Another set of concerns with the new reproductive technologies arises from the feared effects on families and offspring that result from collaborative reproductive transactions with donors and surrogates. The concerns here do not arise when IVF is confined to a married couple, which it now largely is, but they arise from the collaborative arrangements that IVF now makes possible, such as egg and embryo donation and the use of surrogate gestators. The fear is that new genetic, gestational, and rearing combinations, made possible by the technical ability to fertilize eggs externally and transfer them to any physiologically receptive uterus, will confuse the child, confuse the parents, indeed, confuse all of us, and place further stress on the nuclear family.

These arrangements may not be as novel as they first appear. In many respects, they are not drastically different from existing social arrangements that separate genetic, gestational and social parentage. Artificial insemination by donor, adoption, step parentage and various forms of blending families after divorce or death present many of the same concerns, but have been assimilated into the social fabric. Further variations created through egg donation, embryo donation and surrogacy are not radically different and should be treated accordingly. Indeed, in many cases these variations provide genetic or gestational ties with the offspring that do not exist in artificial insemination by donor, adoption or step parentage.

There is a pervasive, though in my view confused, feeling that these arrangements must be harmful to offspring who are born as a result. The problem with this kind of argument is that if it were not for these novel collaborative arrangements, the offspring would never exist. Even if their life is somehow more fraught with psychological difficulties and suffering than the life of the ordinary child, it is the only life possible for them. Prohibiting collaborative transactions thus does not protect the child, for without them the child would never come into being at all. Psychosocial confusion, even genetic bewilderment, is an acceptable price for the offspring to pay in order to exist.

I would argue that couples have a constitutional right to engage in collaborative transactions with donors and surrogates. If married couples (and possibly unmarried persons) have a right to procreate, that right should include the right to make contracts with providers of gametes and embryos and with gestational surrogates, if that is essential to enable them to reproduce and acquire a child of their genes or gestation for rearing. The positive right to procreate thus allows married couples to contract for eggs, sperm, embryos, or surrogates, with the agreement among the parties presumptively settling rearing rights and duties towards the offspring. Unless a tangible harmful impact on offspring or others is demonstrated, such contracts could not be prohibited or limited, though they could be regulated to assure that they are knowingly and freely entered into.

Let us briefly explore these issues with egg and embryo donation and surrogate gestation. It is now possible for women to donate eggs for implantation in other women, and thus have genetic offspring without gestating themselves. At the same time the recipient may gestate and rear a child that is not genetically related to her. Artificial insemination by donor has a well-established niche in infertility treatment for men. The provider of sperm usually gives up all rights and duties with regard to the resulting offspring (which itself may present some problems for the offspring). Is there any reason why women should not also be allowed to donate gametes? Indeed, offspring born of egg donation will have a gestational tie with the mother even though she is not the genetic parent. The same rules that regulate rearing rights and duties to the offspring of sperm donation should apply to egg donation as well: i.e, the agreement between donor and recipient for rearing rights and duties in offspring presumptively controls.

IVF technology allows the extra-corporeal embryo to be implanted into any physiologically receptive uterus, thus making embryo donation possible. Embryo donation is not yet widely practiced, but will occur on a wider scale once the freezing of spare embryos becomes more developed. Embryo donations might also arise from uterine lavage of a blastocyst (an embryo at the 60-100 cell stage) from the uterus of a woman and then transfer of that blastocyst to the womb of another woman. And, of course, laws may develop that mandate donation of unwanted embryos. The question is whether there should be limits or restrictions on embryo donation? Should not the contract between donor and recipient also control in this situation?

It is important that we call this procedure an "embryo donation" rather than "embryo adoption." Use of the term "embryo adoption" smuggles in a hidden value assumption about the nature of the embryo, by analogizing the embryo to an adopted child, an inappropriate analogy, given that it may never implant in the uterus, much less complete the long journey to a term delivery. Embryo donation should be treated like coital reproduction or artificial insemination by donor, where no agency or court review to assure the fitness of parents is required.

A general issue that arises with embryo donation and gamete donation is the question of anonymity and secrecy of the source of the donated embryos and gametes. Can the parties who donate the embryo and the receivers agree among themselves to maintain confidentiality so that the offspring will never know its true genetic origins? Even though the parties agree to confidentiality, the needs of persons born of gamete or embryo donation to know their genetic parents may override the interest of the contracting parties in confidentiality. In this instance the agreement between the reproductive collaborators to maintain a secret would be justly overridden to protect the offspring's interest in knowing his or her genetic roots.

A final point about embryo donation is the possibility of embryo sale. Should people be able to sell the embryo or recoup some of the costs of producing it? Producing excess embryos by IVF is expensive and arduous. Payment beyond the medical costs, however, is objectionable to many persons. Some would argue that embryos should not be sold, and should be treated like organs — hearts, livers, kidneys — which we do not allow to be sold for transplant. But banning payments might interfere with a couple's ability to obtain an embryo, and thus limit their procreative liberty. Unless sale is connected with tangible harm to other persons, the moral or symbolic offense that some people might find in such transactions is not a sound basis for restricting procreative liberty by banning sale of embryos.

Another troubling reproductive transaction concerns gestational surrogacy, the other major collaborative variation that extra-corporeal conception now makes possible. If any extra-corporeal embryo can be transferred to any physiologically receptive uterus for gestation, the gestating woman could choose merely to gestate, and not rear — transferring the child to the persons who provided the embryo in the first place. At least one child from such an arrangement has been born in the United States.

Gestational surrogacy is different from the current practice of "surrogate mothering" that has led to such controversies as the Baby M case recently litigated in New Jersey. That form of surrogacy involves the surrogate's pre-conception agreement to be inseminated, carry to term, and then relinquish the offspring to the father and his partner for rearing. Surrogate gestation, by contrast, involves a pre-implantation agreement with a woman to accept placement of an already created embryo in her uterus for gestation, and then to return it to the genetic parents at birth for rearing.

Surrogate gestation is troubling because of the attitude that it seems to take towards the gestational maternal bond. The willingness to divorce gestation from the usual maternal caring and rearing that occur after birth appears detached and cold, and signifies a willingness to use women as merely gestational vessels.

But gestational surrogacy should also be viewed from the perspective of the woman or couple seeking such reproductive assistance. The strongest demand for such a service would arise from women who are barred by medical factors from gestating their own offspring. A woman may have functioning ovaries, but have had a hysterectomy and not be able to bear a child. Or a woman may have a uterine malformation due to administration of diethystilbesterol to her mother, which makes a successful pregnancy impossible for her. Thus there are legitimate medical reasons why a woman who cannot bear a child, but who is able to produce an egg, may want to engage a surrogate gestator. Some people find these medical needs for a surrogate to be more compelling than reasons of so-called "convenience," where the woman could medically bear the child herself, but for work, life style, leisure and other reasons would prefer not to.

Since hiring a surrogate gestator is an exercise of procreative liberty on the part of the couple, there is a strong case for a constitutional right to employ a surrogate. Prohibition of such arrangements would interfere with the woman's and couple's right to procreate, for there is no other way for them to have offspring of their genes. Harm to the offspring or the surrogate does not appear great enough to justify limitation of the arrangement. Indeed, the main concern appears to be a desire to prevent symbolic harm to deeply-felt notions of motherhood and the importance of the gestational bond.

Treating the gestational bond as something to be manipulated and used for selfish purposes—the willingness to gestate a child and then detach oneself from it—may be distasteful to many people and are legitimate concerns for guiding one's own behavior. But they are not a sufficient basis for public action limiting the procreative choice of willing parties. They should not override the couple's right to procreative liberty and a woman's right to find procreative meaning by serving as a surrogate gestator.

If surrogacy agreements are permitted, they must also be enforced—by money damages if not also by specific performance. Could the surrogate abort or refuse to turn the child over at birth? The argument for allowing the surrogate to renege is weakest when the surrogate is gestating the embryo of another couple. Perhaps she should be free to abort, but if she does, she has breached her contract and destroyed the couple's embryo, and should at least have to pay damages to the couple. One could also argue that she should have to relinquish the child to the genetic parents as the original agreement stated, even if a surrogate who has also provided the egg would be free to keep the offspring. It is the genetic offspring of the hiring couple that is at issue. The surrogate would not have received their embryo for gestation unless she had agreed to relinquish it at birth. Regarding her as a trustee who then must turn over the child should be acceptable, and may even be constitutionally required.

The question of paying surrogates is also controversial. Once again, the argument against payment derive from primarily symbolic distaste at the notion of renting a uterus, and treating women as a uterine function for hire. Beyond the symbolism of hiring gestational vessels is a concern that poor or minority women would disproportionately serve as surrogate gestators. The fear is that poor women would end up bearing the gestational burdens of the middle and upper classes. However, if payment is the only way a couple could produce a child of their own genes, and the surrogate accepts knowingly and freely, there is a strong constitutional argument for permitting payment to surrogates. A prohibition on payment would interfere with this reproductive option, and thus deny couples medically barred from gestating from having and rearing biologic offspring.

THE REIFICATION OF REPRODUCTION

The new reproductive technology is also troubling because of fears that it will lead to Brave New World scenarios and the ultimate reification of reproductive functions. Several issues are conflated in these concerns. One is the fear of technology gone awry and used by government to oppress and enslave. This fear is captured in the frequent reference to Huxley's *Brave New World*, in which children are genetically programmed, produced in laboratories, artificially gestated, and decanted from bottles, already programmed for specific social roles.

A less apocalyptic version of this fear may be expressed as a concern with overtechnologizing intimate human functions. The concern is that we undermine human dignity by subjecting the reproductive process—the very creation of new human beings—to scientific, technical, rational procedures. IVF bombards the ovaries with powerful drugs, invades the body to retrieve eggs, fertilizes eggs under laboratory lights of the laboratory sun and not in the dark recesses of the Fallopian tubes. Yet it is unfair to single out IVF and other new reproductive technologies for these complaints, since similar operations are inherent in science generally, and medical science in particular. Medical science almost always objectifies and manipulates nature.

Futhermore, objectification is inherent in the standard array of infertility treatments now widely accepted. The body is viewed and treated as a kind of technical apparatus to produce gametes and children. Seen in that way, there is nothing distinctive about IVF. It is just an extension of what we do in science, medical science, and infertility therapy generally. Unless we're going to banish all of them, IVF cannot be banned on this ground.

Yet another formulation of the concern with the reification of reproduction focuses on its impact on women. Obviously, only women can ultimately tell us what this impact is. But feminist thinkers are just beginning to address the new reproductive technology, often critically.

Some feminists emphasize the dark side of the new reproductive technology. They deny that it is liberating for women as long as it is women who still gestate, for it binds women to biologic reproductive roles that men escape. True liberation for women would be to reproduce and avoid the burdens of gestation and the concomitant burdens of early child-rearing with which gestation is closely linked.

Furthermore, IVF and its collaborative variations, in focussing on the woman as an object to be made fertile, still assume that a woman's main function is reproductive, and thus reinforce the over-identification of women with biological function. By operating on the woman's and not the man's body, IVF reinforces the notion that the woman is primarily a child-bearer. In this sense, playing more limited or partial reproductive roles as egg donor or surrogate are even more troubling, since they identify the woman with this one aspect of her biologic functioning. Feminists also object to the exploitation and reification of women as gestational vessels that occur with surrogate gestation.

Feminist concerns with the dark side of the new reproductive technology, such as possible exploitation of third world and poor women, and increased male control of reproduction should not be ignored, but I do not believe that they are sufficient to outweigh the benefits to women and men of enhanced choice over fertility. They do remind us, however, of the abuses and problems that are possible, and thus the need to attend to using these techniques carefully.

It seems to me that there is a positive side to the new reproductive technology that feminist criticism has tended to overlook. Extra-corporeal conception seems to promote choice, to promote the autonomy of women (and men) in helping them overcome infertility, which for many women (and men) is a very serious problem. Just being able to have a child and become a parent is a major achievement. These techniques also indirectly support female social roles that might induce infertility, such as postponing childbearing for career or life-style reasons to a time when fertility is greatly lowered.

Extra-corporeal conception also gives women potentially greater control in selecting which embryos will be transferred, thus avoiding the very difficult process that Barbara Katz Rothman discusses in *The Tentative Pregnancy* of undergoing prenatal diagnosis and then possibly choosing abortion to avoid a serious genetic defect in offspring, a very stressful experience. IVF provides a window on the embryo that will eventually enable prenatal diagnosis to occur before implantation, and thus avoid the stresses of abortion for genetic reasons later in the pregnancy.

Finally, IVF technology makes possible new, partial reproductive roles for women. While many women will want to rear their own biologic offspring, some women may find partial reproductive roles as egg and embryo donors and surrogates to be meaningful options that fit best into their life plans.

However one evaluates the potential impact on women, in the short run the new reproductive technologies pose problems that consumers of medical services generally face. IVF reinforces the same problems of male-dominated obstetrics and gynecology that liberal and feminist critics have long decried—the exploitation of women as health care consumers. Questionable uses of hysterectomy, mastectomy, cesarean section and other high-tech obstetrical practices have been justly criticized. Similar concerns may be voiced about the use of IVF, even without its variations, for it is an expensive and stressful experience that often will not produce the baby that the couple so strongly wishes. Yet couples might be misled into thinking that this technology will solve their fertility problems. Most American IVF programs have not yet had a pregnancy, yet many couples are not fully informed of the rather low chance of success. Some IVF programs may thus be exploiting the vulnerability of infertile couples, with the woman bearing most of the burden of physical manipulation. In the short run, the most important issue about the new reproductive technologies for women might be how to assure access to competent, skillful services with fully informed consent.

CONCLUSION

In the final analysis, the new reproductive technologies present a clash between individual autonomy and the social implications of individual procreative choice. In the long run broad social changes could occur from the cumulation of many discrete, individual decisions to use this technology. Yet fear of these long-run consequences should not limit short-run use. Since a basic constitutional right—the right of infertile persons and couples to procreate—is at issue, the state is limited in the measures that it can take to influence the exercise of this right in the private sector.

It may be that many persons exercising their rights will end up changing the values now dominant in society, leading to a new set of procreative values and behavior. But that is the recurring dilemma of liberty in liberal society. The exercise of protected rights may eventually change values and practices throughout the social order. Under the American constitutional scheme, individual discretion over use of the new reproductive technology is protected, even if the exercise of freedom ultimately reshapes the society providing that freedom.

Problems in Commercialized Surrogate Mothering

R. Alta Charo

SUMMARY. Commercialized surrogate mothering is an unworkable arrangement for helping infertile couples to have children. The arrangement requires a woman to undergo artificial insemination, to sustain a pregnancy and to relinquish the child upon birth to the genetic father. During the course of the pregnancy, the arrangement calls for restrictions on the surrogate mother's behavior and authority to make medical decisions concerning herself and the fetus. Such restrictions are unenforceable under contract law, and the usual social mechanisms to induce compliance are absent. Due to the large sums of money involved and the growing industry of surrogate mother brokering, efforts have begun in many state legislatures to regulate the arrangements, and in particular the behavior of the surrogate mothers, in order to increase the predictability and workability of the arrangements. If passed, these state laws could set a dangerous precedent for regulating all women during pregnancy and standardizing the behavior and medical care of pregnant women. Noncommercialized surrogate mothering does not pose these same threats, and is likely to continue for many years to come.

I would like to focus on one aspect of reproductive technologies, namely the so-called "surrogate mothering" whereby women are employed to gestate babies, either genetically their own or someone else's, and to relinquish them upon birth to their genetic fathers. The reason I would like to focus on these women is that their experiences have implications for all pregnant women, particularly with respect to our understanding of the principle of personal autonomy, which underlies our interpretation of procreative liberties.

I find the area of "personal autonomy" very troubling, because it is not well understood in the law. The courts and legislators have not yet heard the hard cases that force clear delineation of views, or allow the public to participate in the debate.* Personal autonomy and procreative liberties are cited as reasons to support and facilitate the use of surrogate mothers, for example, by enacting legislation to recognize, enforce and regulate the contractual arrangements used. I am not convinced, however, that this is either required or workable.

One of the reasons I'm troubled by surrogate mothering is that the whole process is so terribly unmanageable. In the usual pregnancy, a woman and her partner — if she has one — expect to rear the baby soon to be born. Social pressures are brought to bear on the pregnant woman to take care of herself and the growing baby. These pressures come from the woman herself, her family, partner and friends, and encourage her to behave in a certain way during the pregnancy, whether it is to eat well, to refrain from drugs, alcohol and tobacco, to exercise appropriately, or to seek regular medical attention.

In the context of surrogate mothering, the pregnant woman does not intend to keep the baby. Inevitably, this changes her relationship with the child. The usual social pressures are reduced, and commercial pressures are substituted. These pressures consist of the threat to find her liable for damages if the baby is harmed as a result of her actions, or to force her to behave in a way prescribed by the contract. Unfortunately, these remedies are based upon principles of contract law that were designed for commercial transactions, not personal arrangements.

It is a principle of contract law that a contract should be broken whenever it is economically efficient. For example, if I break my contract with you, all I need to pay you are your lost profits on the transaction. I do not pay you for the aggravation I may have caused. Thus, if your profits are less than my savings on another supplier, I am encouraged to break our contract, pay your damages, and form a

---

*Since this paper was written such a case has arisen in New Jersey, popularly known as the "Baby M" case. Mary Beth Whitehead was hired by Mr. and Dr. Stern to have a child for them. She was to be paid $10,000. The Sterns also paid fees to the Infertility Center of New York, which made the arrangements, and covered the medical expenses of Mrs. Whitehead's pregnancy. Upon birth of the child, Mrs. Whitehead found she was unwilling to relinquish her baby.

new contract with the new supplier. I save money, and you are not damaged financially, although you may have been seriously inconvenienced.

This is an unworkable remedy for breach of a surrogate mothering contract. The remedy depends upon an assessment of damages, yet many breaches of behavior, such as smoking tobacco, may lead to no apparent harm to the baby. Further, even if the baby is born with a problem, such as low birth weight, it is exceedingly difficult to connect the specific behavior of the mother with a particular harm to the baby. Smoking does seem associated with low birth weight, but it is unclear how strongly. Babies may have a low birth weight as a result of other factors, either independently, or in combination with smoking. Further, low birth weight itself is not an injury, but merely statistically associated with a variety of infant disorders. How then can we put a price tag on the damages caused by a woman who furtively smokes during the pregnancy?

There is another kind of contract remedy, called "specific performances" to be used when someone breaches a contract for which no replacement can be made, such as a contract for purchase of an original master. In this case, a court can order the party to fulfill the contractual obligation. But this remedy is not used when there is a breach of contract for services, such as a contract to sing at a nightclub, because it is impossible to ensure the quality of the services that will thus be rendered under duress. The same problem arises with surrogate mothering. How can one ensure that the surrogate mother will comply with the court order to follow the contractual limitations on her behavior? Can she be locked up and kept under observation, lest she drink a beer?

Another problem concerns the medical management of the pregnancy. Can we reasonably enforce a contract that purports to take away a pregnant woman's authority to make decisions concerning amniocentesis, abortion, sonography, fetal monitoring or even cesarean sectioning? What are the damages for a refusal to submit to an amniocentesis, particularly if the baby is born free of identifiable disorders? Can we allow a court to order a woman to undergo such a procedure, at some risk to herself and the fetus, upon the request of the sperm donor and on the basis of a contract signed before the woman was examined and shown to be in any need of such a procedure?

Clearly, contract remedies leave much to be desired for enforcing these arrangements, and yet, if surrogate mothering is ever to become big business, it must have some predictability. The result is a growing interest in the regulation of surrogate mothering. By legislating certain behaviors to be required during pregnancy, or by explicitly providing an enforcement mechanism for the contract provisions present, a surrogate could face civil penalties for failure to comply, regardless of the outcome of the pregnancy.

This is not a far-fetched scenario. Legislation has been introduced in over twenty-five states to legalize and in various guises regulate the practice of surrogate mothering. In almost all, the contract is considered enforceable, both with regard to the custody of the baby and to the pregnant woman's behavior. These bills are surprising, as they fly in the face of existing principles of family law, which often disallow contracts exchanging custody for money, even between biological parents, and of contract law, as explained above. Yet the commercial implications of these arrangements, even more than the emotional aspects, drive the legislatures towards a regulated, enforceable arrangement. The emotional pain of losing an expected baby is recognized, but not assuaged, when legislatures require a one month to six month "cooling off" period for mothers who agreed, even during their pregnancies, to give up their babies for adoption. In the surrogate mothering context, however, money changes hands, perhaps as much as $50,000, and the change in attitude among the legislators is evident.

This raises another point, namely the fact that there is an entire industry developing around surrogate mothering. Over a dozen clinics are operating, and they are advertising in papers as disparate as the *International Herald Tribune* and student newspapers, such as *The Columbia Spectator*. These are money-making ventures, aimed at finding surrogates, finding couples willing to risk using surrogates, and overall at creating a market and a legal regime to support it. There is a great deal of money at stake. Fees to the clinic can range up to $50,000 or even $60,000. A small portion of this goes to the woman who will be pregnant for nine months and then relinquish her baby. The bulk will go to the clinic for its services. These include "screening" the surrogate mother. This screening is designed to eliminate women who are unlikely to comply with the contract provisions, thus attempting to head off the need to enforce the contract by any legal mechanism. Screening also includes an evaluation of "emotional health," however that is defined, as well as numerous factors such as looks, education, IQ, interests and other attributes which are more, less or not at all inherited. This screening would not only be sanctioned, but would be required by many states if the legislation introduced to date were to be passed. Few clinics or state bills would require similar screening of the prospective parents, even though at least one is not genetically related to the baby, and would ordinarily require screening before going through an adoption proceeding.

What does all this screening and behavior limitation do to the women employed as surrogates? In essence, it dictates to them the proper demeanor of a woman who intends to be pregnant. Further, as these are commercial ventures issuing standard contracts with standard provisions, women as a group are being evaluated. This is not a development of trivial dimension. In a related area of law, there has been some discussion of the right of children to sue their parents — and in particular, their mothers — for behaviors during pregnancy that resulted in a disorder. Such behaviors include drug and alcohol abuse, or failure to take advantage of amniocentesis or sonography. Recently, one state actually criminally charged a woman with "fetal abuse" for failure to take care of herself properly during pregnancy. At a recent conference of the American Society of Law and Medicine, this topic came under discussion, and I was astounded by the audience reaction. Rather than discuss ways to provide information and nutrition to pregnant women, doctors and lawyers alike began to seriously discuss the possibility of national standards of behavior during pregnancy, with some even talking of regional variations to reflect diverse access to nutrition and health care. This was astonishing, and disturbing, for although it reflected a concern for the fetus, the pregnant woman was viewed largely as a vehicle for the fetus' birth, rather than a whole patient in her own right.

Surrogate mothers, subjected to screening to ensure they are proper vehicles, and to contract limitations on behavior to ensure they carry out their function as gestators, are likely to bear the brunt of any regulations which do develop in this area in the near future, simply because the commercial interests riding on their shoulders and their wombs are so great. But their experiences should function as fair warning to all women. If babies are viewed as articles of commerce, and women as their producers, then the same commercial regulatory philosophies which affect the production of goods will be influencing the way all of us have babies.

It is possible to permit surrogate mothering while avoiding many of these problems, and that is simply to eliminate the commercial brokers. The same was done in the area of adoption, to reduce the abuses of the black-market in babies. Surrogate mothering can never be effectively outlawed, as long as women are willing to undergo at-home artificial insemination or even plain, old-fashioned sexual relations, in order to bear a child for a friend who cannot. Commercial brokers, however, with their commercial contracts and standards of behavior, can be outlawed. This would reduce the drive to widen the market by encouraging couples and women to enter into these agreements and would eliminate much of the pressure on the state legislatures to devise elaborate enforcement mechanisms, with all their potential for one day being extended to all pregnant women.

BIBLIOGRAPHY

Annas, G. 1981. "Contracts to Bear a Child." *The Hastings Center Report* 11(April):22-25.

Annas, G. 1986. "The Baby Broker Boom." *The Hastings Center Report* 16 (June):30-33.

Annas, G. 1986. "Pregnant Women as Fetal Containers." *Hastings Center Report* 16(Dec):13-14.

Brophy, K. M. 1982. "A Surrogate Mother Contract to Bear a Child." *University of Louisville Journal of Family Law* 20:263-291.

Dodd, B. 1982. "The Surrogate Mother Contract in Indiana." *Indiana Law Review* 15:807-830.

Gersz, S. 1984. "The Contract in Surrogate Motherhood: A Review of the Issues." *Law Medicine and Health Care* 12(June):107-114.

Holder, A. 1984. "Surrogate Motherhood: Babies for Fun and Profit." *Law Medicine and Health Care* 12(June):115-117.

Keane, N. and D. Breo. 1981. *The Surrogate Mother*. New York: Dodd.

Koval, E. 1986. *Manufacturing Babies: What Reproductive Technologies Mean to Women.* Canberra: National Women's Consultative Council, Department of Prime Minister and Cabinet.

Krimmel, H. 1983. "The Case Against Surrogate Parenting." *Hastings Center Report* 13:32-37.

Milunsky, A. and G. Annas (eds). 1980. *Genetics and the Law II.* New York: Plenum Press.

Milunsky, A. and G. Annas (eds). 1985. *Genetics and the Law III.* New York: Plenum Press.

Robertson, J. A. 1983. "Procreative Liberty and the Control of Conception, Pregnancy and Childbirth." *Virginia Law Review* 69:405-481.

Robertson, J. A. 1986. "Embryos, Families, and Procreative Liberty: The Legal Structure of the New Reproduction." *Southern California Law Review* 59:939-1041.

Rothman, B. K. 1986. *The Tentative Pregnancy: Prenatal Diagnosis and the Future of Motherhood.* New York: Viking Press, 1986.

Reproductive Technologies
and the Bottom Line

Tabitha Powledge

SUMMARY. Reproductive technologies have turned out to be creatures of the marketplace, a fact we did not foresee. Because of this commercialization, women must be as careful in selecting a clinic as in buying a used car. Where initially it appeared that government would impose test-tube babies and genetic engineering on society, the great irony is that we now look to government to protect us from the Brave New World.

Systematic discussion of social and ethical issues in reproductive technology has been going on at least since the 1960s, and the literature on ethical issues in *in vitro* fertilization is vast and windy.

Some of the issues have faded with time and experience. In 1972, when I first began paying professional attention to IVF, a major concern was whether the process would lead to babies with deformities and other birth defects. Now that many hundreds of test-tube babies are among us, and they seem no different from babies conceived in the usual way, we no longer worry much about the birth defects issue.

I am going to spend very little time discussing the more traditional concerns about IVF. I want instead to turn my attention to an aspect of reproductive technology that is woefully underdiscussed—its commercial prospects and their relation to consumer demand. We need to begin thinking in terms of marketplace influences, not just in connection with IVF, but for all reproductive technologies.

To understand fully how the ethics of reproductive technologies became so intertwined with economics, we need to recall a little history. In the 1970s, the citizens of this country, through their surrogates in the government, made a fateful decision about IVF: they decided NOT to make a decision about it.

We all know that medical research is crucially dependent on government funds for its survival. There are a few private foundations and other groups that underwrite America's medical research, but most research money comes from your taxes and mine, funnelled through a number of government agencies that usually decide how and where it will be spent. That means that the citizenry has in principle some voice in decisions about where the money should go. Occasionally, we even have surprising influence, because Congress holds the purse strings. Sometimes that suits the research establishment. Absolutely everybody is in favor of more money for cancer research, and, more recently, AIDS.

But often researchers and some public groups disagree about which areas medical scientists ought to tackle. By the early 1970s, it was clear that British scientist Robert Edwards was making progress in being able to fertilize eggs in the laboratory, and that there was a good chance that he and his colleague Patrick Steptoe would eventually succeed in bringing actual "test-tube babies" into the world. American researchers wanted to do early embryo research too — not only for reasons of test-tube babies, but also because they wanted to accumulate information about the fertilization process and how the early embryo develops.

So they did what American scientists have been doing for the last couple of decades when they want to research a particular area. They wrote grant proposals to the National Institutes of Health, asking the government for money to underwrite IVF research.

By this time, partly in response to the Supreme Court's landmark decision permitting women to choose abortion, an organized, vociferous right-to-life movement was on the American scene. Its protests had effectively blocked research on fetuses and the early embryo.

In an attempt to resolve this dispute, then come to a decision about whether IVF research ought to be funded with public money, the government resorted to a ploy all of us are familiar with. It appointed a committee. The committee was known as the Ethics Advisory Board. It travelled around the country taking testimony from the public, conducted many discussions, and finally wrote a report, which was published in the spring of 1979.

The report was in some respects a masterpiece of committee work, since in its main conclusions it managed to come down firmly on *both* sides of the issue. Given certain safeguards, it didn't see much ethically wrong with IVF. On the other hand, it also didn't see the work as having a very high priority. As a result, the government to this day has funded no IVF work — not on grounds that it is immoral, but because it has other calls on its funds that it says are more urgent.

At the time of the EAB report, I admired the skill with which the issue had been finessed. The government pleased neither side, and both. It withheld disapproval, but it also withheld money. I was also reasonably happy with its conclusions, since they mirrored my own. Let private developers do this research, I thought. Why spend scarce tax money on it?

Some years later, I am not so sure. I am concerned that, by driving this research out of the public sector and into private hands, we have relinquished control over its development. I did not foresee how much demand there would be for IVF. Despite the expense — $5000 and up per attempt — and the sorry record of success — not more than 20% at even the best clinic — there are said to be as many as 150 IVF clinics in this country alone (and many more elsewhere in the world). IVF is undeniably a phenomenon.

On reflection, of course, I wonder why I didn't guess what would happen. Women have embraced every reproductive technology that's come along. We use birth control methods despite their disadvantages, which range from annoying to lethal. We clamor for prenatal diagnosis whether it's indicated or not, to the point where obstetricians spend a lot of time trying to talk us *out* of it. The heady sense of *really* controlling our reproductive lives has seized us, and we are voting with our feet. And why not? Now, suddenly in the last 20 years, many of us can choose — to forestall our fertility, to circumvent our infertility, even to make some choices about the *kind* of children we have. The word "revolution" is inadequate to describe what is going on, and we are not likely to relinquish it.

Given that mindset, reproductive technologies of all sorts are going to be popular. This is simply a truth about contemporary life, and it should guide our dialogue. For a great many of us, reproductive control is a good that usually outweighs all others. In that context, rarefied discussions of ethical issues frequently seem beside the point, even when they're not. Because infertility is on the increase (due to postponed pregnancies, venereal diseases, and doubtless heaven knows what in our food, air, and water), IVF in particular is likely to grow.

Alas, this new freedom does not result in unalloyed good. IVF is certainly a case in point. Robert Edwards has written interesting memoirs of the early days of IVF in which he makes clear that the women who pioneered the technique suffered terribly. They were forced to disrupt their lives and live under his clinic's regimen for weeks and months at a time, they had to undergo abdominal surgery for egg recovery, and they had to endure disappointment after bitter disappointment at pregnancies that miscarried or, far more often, failed to occur at all.

Somewhat surprisingly, that situation seems to have changed little in the past decade. For a recent example, I refer you to an article in the November 1985 *American Health* magazine, a first-person account of a woman's attempt to create a baby with IVF. On her first trip from upstate New York to the clinic in Norfolk, Virginia, the author is sent home after 10 days because her eggs aren't ripe enough to harvest. On her next visit, which lasts 15 days, embryos are transferred successfully and she actually gets pregnant. But the fetus dies at 21 weeks gestation—and she must carry it, dead, for several weeks, until it is finally aborted. The article concludes with her third visit, which results in another pregnancy. We are not told how that one turned out. This author seems actually to have had a relatively easy time of it. She describes the travails of some of the other women at the clinic, including one who finally succeeded only on her eighth try! Doubtless many disappointed women never make it that far because they run out of hope—or money.

I regard the author's experience as a cautionary tale, but I don't think she does. She's not happy about what she has to go through, but for her it's clearly worth it. The magazine's editors agree. They have titled the article "One Woman's Courage." Neither they nor the author question whether going through such misery for such a small chance of pregnancy makes sense.

What is the role of the clinics themselves in encouraging such a pattern of behavior in their clients? A sign in the Norfolk clinic says, "You never fail until you quit trying." Is this a bit of conventional sunshine folk wisdom, or something more sinister? Let us not forget that these clinics are commercial enterprises. They offer a service for which people pay (and pay handsomely). It is obviously in their interest to encourage persistence, at between $3000 and $7000 a shot.

There is other evidence of the effects of commercial pressures on the way these clinics operate. Observers have raised questions about whether some of the clinics are lying about their success rates. A few have been accused of basing their statistics on the total number of pregnancies they achieve, which means they include positive pregnancy tests that are followed by no discernable pregnancy, and also miscarriages. The important and relevant statistic is, obviously, the ratio of live babies to attempts. The president of the American Fertility Society says the REAL success rate ranges from 20% to 0%, depending on the clinic. And a spokesman for an infertile couples self-help group says, "Many of the clinics do not have any live births to speak of." That is partly a function of the fact that many of the clinics are brand new, of course. But it also reflects the fierce competition for patients.

On reflection, of course, this kind of truth-stretching and exaggeration is only to be expected of a commercial enterprise. The sad truth is that women need to be just as wary and careful and skeptical in selecting an IVF clinic as they are when buying a used car. A time-honored consumer rule applies to both purchases: *caveat emptor*.

If the excess of the marketplace were affecting only IVF, there would perhaps be not much cause for worry. But I think we must face up to the fact that the commercial pressures that are shaping IVF are going to shape other reproductive technologies as well. Let me give you two examples.

It is now possible for some people to choose to have male children. Although parents have been trying to choose their children's sexes for centuries through a variety of theories and practices, and there are dedicated believers in, for example, methods involving timing of intercourse, until recently there was no evidence that any method worked. Now there is one that appears to raise the chance of conceiving a male from 50% to a little over 70% — the so-called Ericsson method in which sperm are centrifuged to separate the male-determining sperm from the female-determining ones, and then inserted through a woman's cervix via artificial insemination.

The Ericsson method is in use at a number of clinics around the world, and although the method is uncertain and not cheap, they do not lack for clients. This, too, is a commercial operation. Just as with IVF, a chance to determine the sex of a child is available to those who can pay for it. But because sex choice is a commercial service, it has come into existence without public debate about its rights and wrongs. The opportunity to choose whether we want our society to go in this direction seems to have passed us by.

My other example comes from the burgeoning field of mammalian genetic engineering. In the past few years, several groups of scientists have made startling progress in their ability to transfer new genes into animal embryos. The techniques are by no means perfected, and will not be for a number of years. Still, scientists can now insert certain genes into an embryo with the assurance that those genes will function in the animal after birth — and that the genes will be passed on to the animal's descendants, where they will also function. Most of this work has been done with mice, but scientists are also forging ahead with applying this work to larger animals, especially pigs and cows. On their immediate agenda is the manipulation of genes for the hormone that controls growth in livestock. Getting control of those genes, the scientists think, will lead to animals that use feed more efficiently and give more milk.

This early work has been supported in part by American taxpayers through such government agencies as NIH and the Department of Agriculture. But private money has flowed into this research as well, and will do so in greater and greater amounts. The profits awaiting those who design better farm animals are stupendous, and it would not surprise me if before long *all* this work is conducted under commercial auspices. Once again we will have lost hold of the purse strings, and missed our chance to reflect thoughtfully about the meaning of these scientific developments for our society.

One major consideration is the implications this work has for our own species. Mice and pigs and cows are mammals, just like us.

We can certainly expect that much of what is learned about genetic engineering in those species will in theory be applicable to us. Especially some years down the road, when mammalian genetic engineering is much more precise and controllable than it is now, are we going to be able to resist trying it on ourselves? Especially if it is in the hands of private developers, and therefore less amenable to social control? How many potential parents with plenty of time and money are going to be able to pass up a chance of choosing some of their children's traits? The temptation will be enormous, and for many irresistible.

The fact that reproductive technologies would turn out to be the creatures of the marketplace was something we simply didn't foresee. Raised on Aldous Huxley's *Brave New World*, and cognizant of the eugenic horrors of the Nazis, we have been led to expect that test-tube babies and human genetic engineering would be imposed on societies through their governments. The great irony is that the very opposite has occurred. We now look to government to *protect* us against the Brave New World.

The NIH committee that has been overseeing the development of therapy for genetic disease has gone to some lengths to explain to the public that this research is *not* human genetic engineering, and that the committee would not consider approving any proposal to engineer human embryos so that their new genes would be passed on to future generations.

I believe these assurances. I think government committees like this one will indeed effectively prevent public money from being spent on human genetic engineering. I also believe that, unless our form of government changes radically, we can dismiss from our minds the idea that our government will impose even the smallest version of a reproductive Brave New World upon us.

But this doesn't mean that we are not moving toward a form of the Brave New World. The recent history of reproductive technologies like IVF and sex choice should be teaching us a great truth: that there is enormous consumer demand for them, and that commercial enterprises are only too happy to meet the demand. With reproductive technologies, we are dealing not with government but with the marketplace, and it looks to me as if we're not going to get to vote.

Technology, Power
and the State

J. A. Mazzeo

SUMMARY. Technical innovations may produce not only the changes they were intended to effect but also lead to consequences which are unexpected and sometimes destructive. There is an intimate relation between technological innovation and political power. Any great advances in reproductive technology are very likely to be controlled and commandeered by the state with all kinds of unforeseeable consequences.

Max Scheler called science "Herrschaft-Wissenschaft," knowledge which gives dominion, thereby separating it from almost any other kind of knowledge we can think of. The question is, to whom does it give dominion?

My whole professional existence has been involved with intellectual history. I think I've been a sensible kind of historian and sensible historians are not prophets. On the other hand, we might hazard one or two guesses. The new reproductive technology—what it is today and what it promises to be in the future—is really without historical precedent. And it would be absurd to hazard more than a few guesses concerning what the future may have in store.

In some respects, the new biological and medical technology resembles a situation which obtained with the appearance of nuclear weapons on the stage of history. The powers that possess nuclear weapons have been able to preserve peace, paradoxically enough, by threatening to use them, and yet not daring to use them. It is a strange paradox, new in the history of warfare and of international conflicts. It is referred to appropriately enough by the acronym MAD: Mutually Assured Destruction. In the same way we may not dare to use the power that biotechnology may place in our hands in the future.

Hegel said that at a certain point quantity becomes quality. You start with dynamite, and then you get TNT and explosives; that's just increasing quantity. But when you proceed to nuclear weapons, you get qualitative change. It introduces a totally new dimension into our problem. This, I think, is what's going to happen, if it hasn't already happened, with biological technology. It's not just a matter of giving some people babies because they happen to want them, or getting rid of babies they don't want, or seeing that the babies are healthy. At the moment, these technologies affect a very small segment of humankind, given the present low rate of efficiency and high expense of the procedures. But if we develop an inexpensive technology, with an implantation success rate of 50%, or sex pre-selection rates of over 90% accuracy, then it is going to affect very many people in the world. Modern technology, biological or physical, seems to have a way of producing new and unexpected problems at the same time that it solves some old ones. In fact, the technological process has a certain kind of autonomy about it, for the new problems require technological fixes—a process which has its own inner determinants, and which seems to escape a very large degree of control. Sometimes the discovery of a rather simple technological innovation may have enormous consequences: for example, the invention of dynamite, the invention of the valve pump, or the pendulum clock, or the escapement mechanism of a spring watch. This last invention made us all clockwatchers.

At the present prices, the new reproductive technology is going to affect only the upper economic classes in only small areas of the world. Once it becomes cheap, then we may have to worry. When a new technology becomes big business, or at least big enough to interest government regulators, then it becomes power. The new technology thus becomes another way in which power expands and institutionalizes itself in society.

Let me offer a simple and crude example of how a seemingly simple biomedical innovation, one well within reach of accomplishment, may have enormous consequences. It should be possible for prospective parents, at some point in the near future, to determine readily the sex of a child they wish to have. If this can be done very efficiently and very cheaply it will have great social and political effects. The mechanism of human reproduction, as it operates naturally, assures in a population a distribution of equal numbers of males and females. Obviously, not in a family, but in a large population. The larger the population, the more nearly equal the numbers should be statistically.

If you suddenly with a pill or with a douche, let us say, or some other easily obtainable means, can pre-determine the sex of a child, then these numbers might get very skewed. Given the widespread preference, in most societies, for boys, governments may have to step in to regulate sex ratios. And such government regulation could only come at the cost of political and reproductive freedoms.

Even this outcome assumes that governments would have rational population policies. But who can be sure that this would be the case? Not too long ago, dictators then taking the world to war assiduously encouraged population growth. They had pronatalist policies. The Hitlers and Mussolinis were out to breed soldiers. And the mothers, who were rewarded as national heroines, were exhorted to be the mothers of warriors. Now, is there any doubt that if Hitler, for example, had possessed a simple way of predetermining the sex of a child, he would have used it?

Similarly, it has been pointed out that if you had a drug which would quickly cure the most intractable forms of psychosis, you would also have a drug which probably could control the behavior of people in ways which, again, a dictator would like to use to consolidate power. Some pessimists foresee a world in which the need for the control of population growth and the need to control the use and distribution of resources will require such great concentrations of power that individual freedoms will become less and less manifest.

Governments may use the new reproductive technologies (against the individual's will) to separate reproduction from the sexual act totally. We have such a phenomenon in insect societies: in the queen bee. One of the science fiction elements before us is that it might also be possible with these technologies to specialize the reproductive functions in society. This, too, has already happened biologically. I refer you to a beehive. Insect societies are controlled and mediated by chemical means. In contrast, humans use words and symbols; our societies are thus mediated by symbolism that requires interpretation. Because insect societies are mediated chemically, they are very efficient. But they are also value-free. The more you control behavior chemically, the more you move towards a society where chemical intervention is the method of choice. Human behavior is already influenced in a limited way with tranquilizers. There are benefits here but also dangers. Indeed, everything that technology brings into being is not unequivocal. It's ambivalent. The results of technological innovation can be used in all sorts of different ways. Insofar as the results increase power, they are not neutral or value-free. We always have to address the questions, What are we going to do with this? Who's going to control it? We must be prepared for all sorts of unforeseen results.

In other words, technology gives us many great benefits, but it does not give them to us in quite the way we would always like to have them. A crude example: technology gives you vacuum cleaners. But the kind of technological society that gives you vacuum cleaners makes domestic labor scarce. So you have to push the cleaner. Still, most people are happy to have vacuum cleaners. With nuclear weapons and now reproductive technologies, the feeling may not be so sanguine.

We frequently hear a self-congratulatory phrase used: how wonderful it is that "modern man" through invention and discovery has acquired such vast power over nature since the seventeenth century. In fact, what we often see, instead, is that relatively few men, by dominating and manipulating nature, wield great political and economic power and in so doing acquire a good deal of dominion over other people.

Each technological advance increases power of one kind or another over natural forces. With each advance, we must ask the same questions: Who will wield this power? For whose benefit? The answers are not always encouraging.

Technology creates power. And the use of power, where it goes, and who exerts it, is fundamentally and finally a political problem. I think, sooner or later, we're going to have to address the political implications of any new technology. Every form of technological innovation I'm acquainted with, historically, has finally been coopted by the state. The state (including our own) claims everywhere dominion over power. It decides how power is distributed, who carries a gun, whether we wage war, whether there is capital punishment. Now the state also enhances itself with technological intervention. That is a grave political and moral danger. As influenced by reproductive technology, the future may have distinct dystopian possibilities.

Prenatal Screening and Discriminatory Attitudes About Disability

Marsha Saxton

SUMMARY. There is a widespread assumption, with the increased use of reproductive technologies, that prenatal screening reduces the incidence of disability and increases our quality of life. However, because of a growing awareness of the social and political implications of prenatal screening, people have begun to challenge these notions about the quality of life and social value of people with disabilities. This paper presents an overview of the issues surrounding prenatal screening of fetuses with intent to abort on the basis of disability. It raises some of the difficult social, political, and personal questions that women, especially prospective mothers, face regarding these issues, and suggests new perspectives for the decision-making process regarding abortion.

"I'm very sorry to tell you, Mrs. Smith, that the fetus you're carrying has been identified as having a defect. Fortunately, we've caught it in time and you can have an abortion."

This statement is a paraphrase of the one that thousands of U.S. women will hear from their doctors this year. With the advent of the new reproductive technology (including blood testing, amniocentesis, and ultrasound), the means to identify a fetus with Down Syndrome, spina bifida, sickle cell anemia, and a growing number of other conditions, allows early detection, usually in the twelfth to sixteenth week of pregnancy. The technologies are heralded by the medical system as a triumph for modern science, a means to control the incidence of disability, and to improve the quality of life for families and society.

217

But there is another point of view, one that challenges the notion that Mrs. Smith will necessarily choose to abort her fetus, and that also contradicts the assumption that the world would be a better place without another disabled person.

I write as a person with spina bifida, the major target of prenatal screening and abortion. I am also a disability rights activist, a former director of a center for persons with disabilities, where I've had the opportunity to meet and get to know closely many hundreds of disabled people. As a disabled person myself, I would like to challenge the rarely examined assumptions that underlie the current trend to screen prenatally and to abort fetuses identified as disabled.

I have been speaking, writing, and leading workshops on this topic for three years.[1] It raises complex emotional, moral, and political questions, but most people have so little information or exposure to the issues of disability that their overriding reaction is: "I've never thought about this!" This response is common to audiences of physicians, nurses, genetic counselors, college professors, parents, and students. (Ironically, disabled people are one of the largest minority groups in the U.S., approximately 40 million people, or over 10 percent of the population, a group that cuts across all gender, ethnic, racial, class, and age lines.)

The assumptions I challenge include these: that having a disabled child is wholly undesirable; that the quality of life for people with disabilities is less than that for others; that we have the means to humanly decide whether some are better off never being born.

These assumptions are pervasive in a society oriented toward rigid standards of beauty and athletic prowess. Disability triggers much fear in our culture. Our pioneer history has led us to revere rugged self-reliance and stalwart productivity; we are not comfortable with the reminder of our vulnerability brought us by disabled people.

The disabled person in our society is the target of attitudes and behaviors from the more able-bodied world that range from gawking to avoidance, pity to resentment, or from vastly lowered expectations to awe. Along with these attitudes, disabled persons confront a variety of tangible barriers: architectural inaccessibility, lack of sign-language interpreters for deaf people, insufficient taped or braille materials for blind persons. In addition, disabled people confront less tangible barriers: discrimination in employment, second-class education, and restricted opportunities for full participation in the life of the community.

As with any kind of oppression, the attitudes are self-perpetuating, and the stereotypes are reinforced in the popular media. The isolation of disabled persons limits the larger culture's exposure to their life experiences, needs, and common humanness. A child's natural curiosity and inquisitiveness in encountering a disabled person for the first time is often met with a parent's embarrassed, "Hush, don't ask and don't stare." This child's simple wonder is thus replaced with mistrust and fear, to be handed down the generations. As recently as the 1950s, laws remained on the books in some states prohibiting the public presence of persons "diseased, maimed, mutilated or in any way deformed so as to be an unsightly or disgusting object." This fear of vulnerability, this flight from physical limitation (perhaps from death) is at the root of such phenomena as the Eugenics Movement in the early 1900s. By 1937, 28 states had adopted Eugenics Sterilization laws aimed at persons with epilepsy, mental retardation, mental illness, and other kinds of differences where "procreation was deemed inadvisable." Such attitudes are still with us.

Where do these attitudes come from? Many women are familiar with the widespread advice physicians give to parents who give birth to a disabled child: "Put him away in a home with others like himself." Institutionalization is an outgrowth of the assumption that neither the parents nor the community could cope with the child at home. Such an assumption becomes a self-fulfilling prophecy: the family, friends, and community are never exposed to the child and its actual needs, so dreaded fantasies reinforce stereotypes. The child, as a result of being institutionalized, does indeed become a social outcast, ill-prepared to cope with community life, exhibiting many of the asocial behaviors and extreme dependencies which the parents had feared.

How do the oppressive attitudes about disability affect the woman considering prenatal screening? Very often prospective parents have never faced the issue of disability until it is raised in relation to testing. What comes to the minds of most prospective parents at the mention of the term "birth defects"? Our exposure to disabled children has been so limited because of their isolation that most people have only stereotyped views, which include images derived from telethons and displays on drugstore counters soliciting our pity and loose change. The image of a child with Down Syndrome elicits an even more intense assumption of eternal parental burden.

The fear that a handicapped child will be a burden seems to be a prominent issue in the decision to abort. How much reality is there to the "burden of the disabled"?

In a popular women's magazine, I read "a young mother's story" about a family with a severely disabled child. The mother's description of her struggle to care for the child and another nondisabled sibling in their suburban home struck me: this woman, the sole caretaker of the children, had no assistance from her working husband and none also from any extended family, or from neighbors, or community. She mentioned no contacts with associations for parents in her situation, or community services, only contacts with the child's physician. Of course, she was lonely and overwhelmed; she was isolated by the limitations of the nuclear family.

I do not mean to imply that it's easy to raise a disabled child, emotionally or logistically, even where there *are* additional resources and support systems. But I do suggest that the common assumptions which place the primary blame for the parents' difficulties on the child's disability vastly distort the picture.

A few years ago I attended a weekend conference for families involved in a program called "Project IMPACT" (Innovative Matching of Parents And Children Together). This program arranges adoptions for "hard to place" children, many with multiple handicaps such as mobility impairments, hearing or vision loss, or mental retardation. Having previously led workshops and support groups for parents of disabled children, I was familiar with the many issues such families face: feelings of guilt, and resentment at the limited social services and practical resources. I arrived curious about the parents I would meet there. Unlike most of the parents I had counseled, these parents had *chosen* to raise disabled children. I met with about forty of these families and learned of their experiences and feelings, their ways of dealing with their situations. What struck me was that the usual feelings of "burden" seemed consistently to be replaced with a sense of challenge to find solutions, to meet with others who had found new answers to this or that question, or to share what they had learned. Absent was the attitude "Why me?" or "What did I do to deserve this?" so common among the many other parents of disabled children. To the IMPACT parents, their disabled children served as a source of enrichment, growth, challenge, and joy.

I was reminded of the many mothers of disabled children whom I have seen grow and change over the years. One in particular, Emily, had struck me as especially timid and passive when she first came for training and support to advocate for her disabled child's rights in the school system. Through the course of the work she did on behalf of her child in the six years I knew her, she blossomed, she grew, she became a leader of others, she became triumphant in her new strength as a fighter against discrimination. Her disabled child, originally perceived as the source of her difficulty, had become the impetus for her transformation.

So often *disability is perceived as the problem*, when in fact the disability becomes *the arena* to play out deep seated distress, disappointment, losses. When seen with clarity and infused with adequate support, the disability becomes the motivation to re-evaluate old attitudes and formulate a more meaningful and satisfying life.

Another of the stereotypes affecting prospective parents concerns "suffering"; it is assumed that disabled persons' lives are filled with pain.

In my work as a therapist, trainer, and former director of a counseling center, I've gotten to know closely the lives of severely disabled people: people with quadriplegia, multiple sclerosis, muscular dystrophy, cerebral palsy, people who are blind or have hearing impairments, "hidden" chronic diseases such as epilepsy and diabetes. Just as the larger population, some of these individuals experience considerable difficulty in their lives while others do fine, have jobs, and enjoy a full and satisfying life with their friends and families. Most disabled people have told me with no uncertainty that the disability, the pain, the need for compensatory devices and assistance can produce considerable inconvenience, but that very often these become minimal or are forgotten once the individual makes the transition of living everyday life. But it is the discriminatory attitudes and thoughtless behavior that make life difficult. These are the source of the real limits; the oppression, the architectural barriers, the pitying stares or frightened avoidance, the unaware assumptions that "you couldn't do the job," couldn't order for yourself in a restaurant, couldn't find a mate or direct your own life. The *oppression*, as I have heard many other disabled people say, in one way or another, is what's disabling about disability.

There is no doubt that there are disabled people who "suffer" from their physical conditions. There are even those who may choose to end their lives rather than continue in pain or with severe limitations, but this is obviously also true for nondisabled people who suffer from emotional pain and limitation of resources. As a group, people with disabilities do not "suffer" any more than any other group or category of humans. Our limitations may be more outwardly visible, our need for help more apparent, but like anybody else, the "suffering" we may experience is primarily a result of not enough human caring, acceptance, and respect.

Often when I speak at conferences, a participant will comment that they know of a disabled person who has suffered greatly: a child who has become the guinea pig in a series of experimental operations to keep her alive; a middle-aged person in constant pain from cancer; an aged person on life support machines. "Wouldn't these people be better off dead?" is the question the participant is really asking.

In advocating that the disabled fetus be allowed to live (and be accepted and loved as any child), I also advocate that terminally ill people be allowed to die, and with dignity. It is often the case that aging, dying individuals in medical institutions are suffering as much from the loss of power over their own affairs, disorientation at being away from home, and objectification as a diseased body, as they are from their illness. Regarding these extreme cases of suffering, the point is that here again, we attempt to *control* life from a vantage point distorted by our own confusions and erroneous attitudes.

I advocate that people be allowed to live and die according to their *own* volition. Above all I challenge the assumption that we as a culture and as individuals have the essential and profound clarity to assess the quality of life for others and to humanely determine their fate.

The medical system wishes to fix, to cure, to control, to perfect, reinforcing the ideal and the possibility of the "perfect baby." Physicians exert strong influence over consumers regarding prenatal screening and they often function as the primary counsel to prospective parents. Because physicians are under pressure to encourage prenatal screening and even abortion out of fear of malpractice suits, they may lobby for enforced screening and will certainly encourage more screening. But physicians, by the very nature of their work, often have a distorted picture of disability. By working in hospitals, with sick people, doctors generally see only those cases of disability where there are complications, where patients are poorly managed, or patients in terminal stages. Many physicians never have the opportunity to see disabled individuals living independently, productively, enjoyably.

If I could counsel to a woman considering prenatal screening with possible intent to abort a disabled fetus, I would ask her: Was she satisfied that she had sufficient knowledge about disability, an awareness of her own feelings about it so that she could make a rational choice? Did she personally know any disabled adults or children? What was she taught about disability by adults when she was young? Was she aware of the distorted picture of the lives of disabled people presented by the posters, telethons, and stereotyped characters in the literature and media? I would ask her to consider the opportunities for herself in taking on the fears and prejudice, the expectations and pressures of her family and friends.

I would suggest that the major factors to consider in decision making are the *resources* of the parents, the family, the community, to care for and love and encourage the child to its fullest potential, and that accurate assessment of those resources can come only with greater clarity about the real nature of disability. By confronting our human vulnerability rather than denying or attempting to take flight from it, we achieve the deepest experience of our humanness.

We will most likely never achieve the means to eliminate disability: our compelling and more profound challenge is to eliminate oppression. Our achievement of acceptance of all people with differences will bring the greatest enhancement of the quality of our lives.

NOTE

1. "Born and Unborn: Implications of the Reproductive Technologies for People with Disabilities" by Marsha Saxton, in *Test Tube Women: What Future for Motherhood*? edited by Rita Arditti, Renate Duelli-Klein and Shelly Minden. Boston: Routledge and Kegan Paul, 1984.

BIBLIOGRAPHY

"The Implications of 'Choice' for People with Disabilities" by Marsha Saxton, in *Women Wise*, The N.H. Feminist Health Center Quarterly, Winter 1984.

Eugenics:
New Tools, Old Ideas

Ruth Hubbard

SUMMARY. Prejudices against people who have noticeable disabilities have resulted in needless social and economic barriers to their participation in society. In Germany under the Nazis, a movement for eugenics, or "racial hygiene," led to the sterilization and, later, the elimination of people with particular mental or physical disabilities. In the United States, earlier in the century, the eugenics movement produced compulsory sterilization laws. At present, physicians and scientists are developing techniques for prenatal diagnosis of increasing numbers of inherited diseases and disabilities, although more babies and children are needlessly disabled because of poverty and accidents than for genetic reasons. Such prenatal tests are being hailed as progress, yet their availability is once again turning pregnancy into a medical event and confronts women with decisions and choices that can be extremely difficult.

A eugenic ideology prevails in this and other countries that finds its political expression in a neglect of the needs and civil rights of people with disabilities. As a result, people who have a disability confront unnecessary and arbitrary barriers to education and employment, which make it difficult for them to live ordinary lives. These kinds of difficulties, as well as ignorance and fear of disability, make many people feel that it would be impossible for them to raise a child with a disability. Such prejudices and the resulting problems that people with disabilities face lend a sense of urgency to the development and use of techniques for detecting genetic or developmental disabilities of the fetus during pregnancy so as to prevent the birth of disabled infants.

225

To avoid any possible misunderstanding, I want to state at the outset that I support a woman's right to abortion, whatever her reasons, but I also think that eugenic reasons for abortion are different from not wanting to be pregnant at all. In fact, recent research has shown that abortions of wanted pregnancies, because the fetus has been diagnosed to have a disability, can be very distressing even to women who are not opposed to abortion on principle (Rapp 1984; Rothman, 1986). Therefore I think that the eugenic thrust is far from liberatory for pregnant women and for the rest of society and that the technologies of prenatal diagnosis have other, more problematic, effects than merely opening choices.

WHAT IS EUGENICS?

The term *eugenics* was coined by Francis Galton in 1883. Galton was an upper-class Englishman, a cousin of Charles Darwin, and a mathematician who in a sense invented statistics. The word is derived from the Greek for "well-born." What Galton (1883) was looking for was "a brief word to express the science of improving the stock, which is by no means confined to questions of judicious mating but which, especially in the case of man [sic] takes cognizance of all the influences that tend in however remote a degree to give the most suitable races or strains of blood a better chance of prevailing speedily over the less suitable than they otherwise would have had" (24-25). So his intent was clear.

More than a decade earlier, Galton (1869) had written a book called *Hereditary Genius* in which he set out to answer the question why getting honors at Cambridge University runs in families, as does being a judge, statesman, divine, literary man or scientist. He decided that these capacities were biologically inherited and that Britons were particularly well endowed in this regard, though note that the pattern of inheritance he observed operates only in the male line. Galton realized that eugenics can be implemented in two ways: positive eugenics, that is, getting the better stocks, as he called them, to have more children; and negative eugenics, which means restraining the less desirable elements from reproducing. (Among such less desirable elements were what he called the mentally ill and feeble-minded as well as habitual paupers and criminals.)

The assumption that this is a way to improve society is based on the simplistic, though not uncommon, notion that a society's characteristics merely reflect the sum total of traits of the individuals that compose it. It is interesting that as late as 1941, while Nazi eugenics was in full swing, the distinguished biologist Julian Huxley (1941) argued that it was crucial for society that mental defectives (his term) not have children. But he also pointed out, and this is looking forward to where we are now, that the most effective way to erase mental defects, which he assumed to be almost always hereditary, would be not merely to prevent people with such "defects" from having children but to be able to predict who among "normal" people might be carriers of "defects" and prevent them, too, from having children.

So, prenatal genetic screening was in the cards long before there was a way to do it effectively. The reason why Huxley saw a need for genetic screening is that most of the so-called "inherited defects" are what is called recessive. What this means is that if a person has a gene for the disease on only one of the appropriate pair of chromosomes (and all human chromosomes, except the so-called sex chromosomes of males, come in pairs), s/he shows no symptoms and therefore does not know it is there. To exhibit the trait, a person must have the corresponding gene on both chromosomes. People who have only one gene for a recessive trait, which they therefore do not manifest, are called carriers. If a carrier of a particular, harmful trait (who, of course, does not know that s/he is a carrier) has a child with another person who also does not manifest the trait, but carries it, their child has one chance in four of manifesting the trait in question. Most inherited diseases and disabilities are of this sort, which means that they cannot be eliminated by preventing merely the people who have the problem from having children, since the gene is diffused widely among the "carriers" in the population. The people who manifest the disease are just the tip of the iceberg.

The eugenics movement in the United States took off essentially from Galton's assumptions. In 1910, a Eugenics Record Office was established in Cold Spring Harbor under the direction of Charles Davenport, a biologist, who had previously been on the faculties of Harvard and the University of Chicago. He hired a bevy of field workers who accumulated large numbers of pedigrees of so-called mental and social defectives on Long Island and in New York City.

The work of the Eugenics Record Office and the broader eugenics movement in the United States had two legislative outcomes: compulsory sterilization law and the Immigration Restriction Act of 1924. The first compulsory sterilization law was enacted by Indiana in 1907, and by 1931 some 30 states had such laws on their books. These laws were intended for so-called sexual perverts, drug fiends, drunkards, epileptics and "other diseased and degenerate persons" (Ludmerer 1972:92). Although most of these laws were not enforced, by January 1935 some 20,000 people in the United States had been forcibly sterilized, nearly half of them in California. In fact, the California law was not repealed until 1980, and eugenic sterilization laws are still on the books in some 20 states.

The Immigration Restriction Act, which I won't go into here, was instituted to limit the proportion of poor immigrants from southern and eastern Europe so as to give greater predominance to Americans of British and north-European descent.

NAZI EUGENICS

I want now to turn to Nazi eugenics because it is often misrepresented and therefore usually misunderstood. Nazi eugenic policies were not the creations of ignorant and evil politicians. The German eugenics program was constructed and implemented by physicians and scientists, mainly geneticists, anthropologists, and psychiatrists, who were professors at major universities, heads of departments, writers of established textbooks in their fields, and heads of research institutes. They were joined by legal experts, also at the top of their profession.

In Germany, eugenics was called racial hygiene, and was looked upon as a program in public health. What distinguished Germany from Britain or the United States was that the political climate under the Nazis made it possible for scientists, physicians, and jurists to put together and implement programs of racial hygiene that could not be put forward elsewhere, and they knew that. For example, Eugen Fischer, Director of the Kaiser Wilhelm Institute for Anthropology, Human Genetics, and Eugenics in Berlin from 1927 to 1942, looking back over the history of German racial hygiene wrote in 1943: "It is special and rare good luck when research of an intrinsically theoretical nature falls into a time when the general world view appreciates and welcomes it and, what is more, when its practical results are immediately accepted as the basis for governmental procedures" (Müller-Hill 1984:64; my translation). Historians of the Nazi period, such as Müller-Hill (1984) and Proctor (1988), who have been examining different aspects of the Nazi eugenics movement, have emphasized that it is not true, as has sometimes been claimed, that these scientists were perverted by Nazi racism. As Proctor has pointed out, it was largely medical scientists who invented racial hygiene in the first place.

Racial hygiene initially was developed to eliminate the same kinds of people whom the British and American eugenicists worried about. It was not directed against Jews, Gypsies, Gays, and eastern Europeans, the kinds of people who come to mind when we think of the Nazi persecution and extermination programs. That came later. Initially, racial hygiene was designed to eliminate "hereditary pathology." To this end, in July 1933, barely six months after Hitler came to power, the government passed the eugenic sterilization law which established local Genetic Health Courts, presided over by one lawyer and two physicians, whose ruling could be appealed to similarly constituted Supreme Genetic Health Courts. But let me point out at once that only one or two percent of lower court rulings were ever reversed at the higher level.

The Genetic Health Courts could order sterilization on the grounds that someone had a "genetically determined disease," such as "inborn feeble-mindedness, schizophrenia, manic-depressive insanity, hereditary epilepsy, Huntington's disease, hereditary blindness, hereditary deafness, severe physical malformation, and severe alcoholism" (Müller-Hill 1984:32; my translation). Physicians were expected to report such patients and their close relatives to the nearest local health court, and would be fined if they failed to do so. When physicians raised the objection that such a requirement invaded the doctor-patient relationship and undermined confidentiality, the authorities replied that this was a public health measure, no different from requirements to report infectious diseases, such as TB or scarlet fever, or births and deaths.

By the beginning of World War II, in 1939, some 300,000 to 400,000 people had been sterilized, with a mortality rate of about

1/2% — about 1,500 to 2,000 deaths. A German friend has told me the following anecdote: her mother's sister had epilepsy. During the entire Nazi period, the family lived in terror that this woman might have an attack in a public place where it would be reported, in which case she and all her close relatives would be subject to sterilization. My friend pointed out that the program was not as efficient as its promulgators wished, but given present ways of keeping track of people by means of computerized data banks, such a policy could now be implemented much more effectively.

The sterilization program in Germany slowed down around the beginning of the war, at which time the euthanasia program came to the fore. This program, too, was not just a mindless, arbitrary excess: it was a carefully designed program of "selection and eradication," as it was officially called, of people who were deemed not fit to live. Actually, already in 1935 plans were initiated for the "destruction of lives not worth living." The phrase, "the destruction of lives not worth living," comes from the title of a book published much earlier, in 1920, by a professor of psychiatry and director of the psychiatric clinic at Freiburg, Alfred Hoche, and Rudolf Binding, a professor of jurisprudence at the University of Leipzig. In translation, it is entitled *The Release for Destruction of Lives not Worth Living.* (In 1985, during the renewed search for Dr. Mengele, the physician who had supervised the selection of victims for research at Auschwitz, newspapers quoted his son as saying that Mengele never changed his mind about the propriety of his scientific work and that he continued to talk about "worthless lives.")

Again, it is important to underline that initially the euthanasia program was directed not against Jews, Gypsies, and other victims of the later extermination programs, but against inmates of psychiatric hospitals and against children institutionalized for mental and physical disabilities — at first only children under three years, later also older children. Indeed, initially, Jews were specifically excepted as not worthy of euthanasia. For this initial "euthanasia" program the gas chambers were developed, and the victims were given soap and towels and told that they were about to have a shower in order to get them to walk into the gas chambers on their own — all practices later used in the extermination camps. This is also where the different kinds of lethal gas were tested: carbon monoxide, cyanide, and eventually Cyclon B, which came to be the gas of choice in the concentration camps. Everything was tried out here, including special crematoria for the mass disposal of victims after they had been gassed.

The euthanasia program was instituted as the war began and some people have speculated that perhaps it could not have been implemented if it were not for the general dislocation of the war. Be that as it may, it began with the compulsory registration by pediatricians of all children with Down Syndrome, microencephaly and various physical deformities who were in their care. A team of medical experts was appointed to go over these forms and, without seeing the children, mark each form with a plus or minus sign. Children whose form was marked plus were transferred to one of a number of institutions where they were killed. Initially, as I said before, the program was directed at children under three years old, by 1941 also at older children with disabilities, but by 1943 healthy Jewish children were included. In 1939, the selection of adult inmates of psychiatric institutions for euthanasia began as well. By September 1941, over 70,000 patients had been killed at some of the oldest and most respected psychiatric institutions in Germany. Relatives were informed that their family member had died suddenly of one or another natural cause and had been cremated for reasons of public health. But rumors could not be contained and the euthanasia program aroused protests, especially from the church. The killing of hospital inmates therefore was virtually ended by 1941, and replaced by the mass exterminations in concentration camps that we all know about. Similarly, when the program of individual, one-by-one sterilizations was stopped, it was converted to mass sterilizations carried out in concentration camps, which included experiments to test different doses of X-rays and various chemicals.

PRENATAL DIAGNOSIS

What is the relevance of this gruesome history to the present-day uses of genetic counseling and prenatal diagnosis? Some people argue vehemently that there isn't any. But I see a connection that I can sum up best by a quote from Hannah Arendt's (1977:279) book on Eichmann: who has "any right to determine who should and should not inhabit the world?'' That is what I want to reflect on in these last pages.

As I said before, I firmly believe in every woman's right to terminate her pregnancy, whatever her reasons. I do not think anyone should have to bear or raise a child if she is unwilling or feels unable to do so. So why am I comparing the eugenic practices of the Nazis with present-day programs of prenatal diagnosis? It is because I want to emphasize the thread that I believe links the Nazi's eugenic practices and ours: the belief that disability is unmitigated disaster, that we would be better off if people with disabilities did not exist. This and the unnecessary limitations imposed on people with special needs are what make women, and men, feel that they owe it to themselves, their families, their future child and perhaps to society as a whole not to bring a child with special needs into the world.

Now as then, scientists and physicians are in a position to provide the means with which to act on the eugenic prejudices of the society which they share. And once a technique exists to identify a fetus that will be born with a particular disability, individual women and families become responsible for acting out these prejudices. If a test is available and a woman doesn't use it, or completes the pregnancy although she has been told that her child will have a disability, the child's disability is no longer an act of fate. She is now responsible; it has become her fault. In this liberal and individualistic society, there may be no need for eugenic legislation. Physicians and scientists need merely provide the techniques that make individual women, and parents, responsible for implementing the society's prejudices, so to speak, by choice.

This society acts as though people with disabilities did not exist, by not enforcing their rights to equal access, employment and housing, and by not providing for their special needs. Under these circumstances, scientists and physicians can take pride in providing means of prenatal diagnosis so that such people need not be born. The possibilities for expanding the technology are great, so that with time it will be possible to detect more and more, rarer and rarer disabilities prenatally. Yet we have no procedures by which to decide, as a society, ''who should and who should not inhabit the world. '' It is up to individual professionals, operating within professional settings, to decide which tests to develop. And once the means to avoid bearing a child with a particular disability are available, women who have medical and financial access to that so-called choice may not feel entitled to refuse.

Let me be clear: I assume that most parents would like to have healthy children. Its health and its sex usually are the first things we ask about when the baby is born. The question is how best to attain that. At present in the United States, the main predictors of disabilities and diseases of newborns and young children are not genetic. They are poverty and extreme youth, or age, of the mother (Rodov and Santangelo, 1979). Indeed, poverty and extreme youth often go together. If we, as a society, are concerned to produce as healthy babies as we can, we should be putting our energies into meeting women's needs for education, healthful home and work environments, good nutrition and prenatal care (Task Force on Prevention of Low Birthweight and Infant Mortality, 1985). It makes no sense to be putting resources into learning how to diagnose relatively rare diseases so as to prevent the babies who have them from being born, while we permit potentially healthy babies to be disabled for reasons that are well-understood and preventable. But it makes sense to put greater resources into learning about the major disabling diseases with an eye to preventing, ameliorating, or curing them. At the same time, we need to make it possible for people who have disabilities to get what they need in order to live fulfilling lives.

The fear of disabilities and revulsion against people who have them are undermining the realistic assessments we feminists made when we insisted on "taking our bodies back." So, here we are taking our pregnant bellies back to the doctor's office, so he (and now occasionally she) can reassure us that our baby will be "normal." It would not be so bad if physicians advocated the use of prenatal diagnosis only for the rare woman who has a reason to be concerned that her baby may inherit a specific, serious health problem because of her own or her partner's family history. But we live in a society in which economic investments in technology are amortized by marketing the techniques as widely as possible. So now, because the tests exist, every pregnant woman in California *must* be offered screening for neural tube defects; every pregnant woman over 35, who can afford to pay for the tests and for the abortion she may subsequently decide to have, is offered screening for Down Syndrome. And so it goes: Tay-Sachs screening for Ashkenazi Jews, sickle cell screening for Blacks, and more.

We in the United States hold up pluralism and diversity as ideals, even through we do not always live by them, when it comes to race, ethnicity, religious beliefs, and cultural differences. But we live with an unspoken and unexamined healthism and able-ism that puts the differences arising from disability beyond the pale. The media ignore people who are disabled or portray them in one of two ways — heroic or pitiful. But people with disabilities do not fit stereotypes any better than the rest of us do. They, too, are individuals with different strengths and weaknesses, capabilities and deficiencies.

When I became concerned about the effects of prenatal diagnosis on pregnant women and on society, I hardly knew anyone with a noticeable disability. I had made no effort to know such people and, no doubt, I had even avoided doing so. Through my work, I have now met quite a number of people who have disabilities and have become friends with several of them. Most of the time when I am with them, I do not think about their disability. But when I do, what strikes me most is the flexibility of human beings, the variety of ways in which people cope with different challenges and needs. And I am struck by the extent to which many of us who are, so to speak, healthy and normal (always a matter of degree) let our emotional and physical resources atrophy because we do not use them. People who differ from us because of a disability have as much to teach us as people who have grown up in different cultures — and we them. Raising a child with a disability can be painful and enjoyable, debilitating and enriching, like raising any child, only perhaps more so. True, some disabilities can be so devastating and disfiguring that they do not call forth our strengths, but overwhelm us. These are extremely rare, and with our present ways of living, we are more likely to encounter them because a loved one has a near-fatal accident than because s/he is born that way. We do ourselves an injury, as individuals and as a society, if we let fear of difference tempt us to decide "who should and who should not inhabit the world" because it is hubris to pretend that we have the knowledge and foresight to make such judgments well. Our job, as a society, is not to weed out those who do not conform to particular standards, but to make it possible for different kinds of people to live their lives as fully as they can.

BIBLIOGRAPHY

Galton, F. 1869. *Heredity Genius*. London: Macmillan.

Galton, F. 1883. *Inquiries into Human Faculty*. London: Macmillan.

Huxley, J. 1941. "The Vital Importance of Eugenics." *Harper's Monthly* 163(August):324-331.

Ludmerer, K. M. 1972. *Genetics and American Society: A Historical Appraisal*. Baltimore: Johns Hopkins University Press.

Müller-Hill, B. 1984. *Tödliche Wissenschaft: Die Aussonderung von Juden, Zigeunern and Geisteskranken, 1933-1945 (Deadly Science: The Elimination of Jews, Gypsies, and the Mentally Ill, 1933-1945)*. Reibek bei Hamburg: Rowohlt.

Proctor, R. 1988. *Racial Hygiene: Medicine under the Nazis*. Cambridge, MA: Harvard University Press.

Rapp, R. "XYLO: A True Story." Pp. 313-328 in *Test-Tube Women: What Future for Motherhood?* edited by R. Arditti, R. Duelli Klein and S. Minden. London: Pandora Press.

Rothman, B. K. 1986. *The Tentative Pregnancy: Prenatal Diagnosis and the Future of Motherhood*. New York: Viking.

Rudov, M. H. and N. Santangelo. 1979. *Health Status of Minorities and Low-Income Groups*. Washington, D.C.: U.S. Government Printing Office HEW Publication No. (HRA) 79-627.

Task Force on Prevention of Low Birthweight and Infant Mortality. 1985. *Closing the Gaps: Strategies for Improving the Health of Massachusetts Infants*. Boston, MA: Dept. of Public Health.

Women and
Reproductive Technologies:
A Partially Annotated Bibliography

Donna M. Cirasole
Joni Seager

SUMMARY. This bibliography is a resource for further information about Women and Reproductive Technologies. The references are categorized as General Information, Law and Policy Considerations, and Information about Specific Technologies. It also lists periodicals, organizations, and other bibliographies relating to this subject and is current through March 1986.

PREFACE

Amniocentesis, *in vitro* fertilization, eugenics, surrogate motherhood, abortion—each of these processes, techniques, ideas, is part of the phenomenon of reproductive technology. Reproductive technologies have wide-ranging implications for women, as well as for family life and society as a whole. This bibliography lists some of the available literature on the facts and effects of such technologies. Many of the selections examine their ethical, political, and legal ramifications. Several related topics, such as contraception and family planning, genetic screening, and environmental reproductive hazards, have not been discussed here.

The first part of this bibliography deals with general issues relat-

---

Many of the references in this section were found in: Doris Sutterley and Elizabeth Schachne (compilers). *Health Care, Medical Ethics, and Reproductive Issues: A Working Bibliography, 1977-1985*. Princeton University: Program in Women's Studies, 1985.

ing to reproductive technology. Part II includes law and policy considerations. It focuses on the legal rights of the mother and of the fetus. Other political and legal issues are also discussed.

Part III distinguishes the individual techniques. The section on fetal testing includes information about amniocentesis and other techniques. It also deals with the use of fetal testing for abortion decisions. Abortion is discussed in general and in terms of its uses for sex preselection and in cases of disability.

Sex preselection is also a possible consequence of the techniques described in the next section: Technologies Affecting Conception. In this section, information about the techniques of *in vitro* fertilization and artificial insemination is presented. The process of surrogate motherhood is also addressed.

The last section in Part III includes information about sterilization and contraception. A subsection on Depo-Provera, a long-acting hormonal contraceptive, is included.[1]

Part IV lists additional resources. These are grouped as periodicals, organizations, and bibliographies.

Many people assisted in the preparation of this bibliography. I would especially like to thank Dr. Ruth Perry and Cynthia Brown of the MIT Program in Women's Studies and Nachama Wilker and the other members of the Women and Reproductive Technologies group of the Committee for Responsible Genetics in Boston for their assistance.

I. GENERAL INFORMATION

A. Books

Arditti, Rita, Renate Duelli Klein and Shelley Minden, eds. *Test-Tube Women: What Future for Motherhood?* Boston: Pandora Press, 1984.

> A collection of essays discussing the effects of reproductive technology: Are they liberating or oppressive? Consideration of outside controls over women, including technological interference, legal regulations, and social pressures.

Bennett, Neil G., ed. *Sex Selection of Children*. New York: Academic Press, 1981.

A comprehensive ethical and sociological analysis of the possible effects of sex selection of children. Consideration of the effects on parents, children, developed and developing countries, etc.

See especially chapter 3, "Sex Selection through Amniocentesis and Selective Abortion" and chapter 5, "Decision Making and Sex Selection with Biased Technologies."

Bernard, Jessie. *The Future of Motherhood*. New York: The Dial Press, 1974.

See especially chapters 13 and 14 on "Medical, Pharmacological, and Psychological Technologies" and "The Politics of Motherhood."

Blank, Robert. *The Political Implications of Human Genetic Technology*. Boulder, CO: Westview Press, 1981.

Boston Women's Health Book Collective. *The New Our Bodies, Ourselves*, 3rd edition. New York: Simon & Schuster, 1985.

See Chapter 17: "New Reproductive Technologies." Ruth Hubbard, with Wendy Sanford.

Summaries of donor insemination, surrogate motherhood, *in vitro* fertilization (IVF), sex preselection, and future possibilities (artificial parthenogenesis, egg fusion, and cloning). Discussion of issues of invasiveness and manipulation, sexual and economic discrimination, long-range goals, society's valuation of fertility, and who will profit.

Corea, Gena. *The Mother Machine: Reproductive Technologies from Artificial Insemination to Artificial Wombs*. New York: Harper & Row, 1985.

Definition of Foreground as the surface reality—in this case, technology itself—and Background as the underlying truths. Consideration of the effects of social and political context on women's choices: our motivation, society's valuation and exploitation of women, men as the dominant class.

Daly, Mary. *GYN/Ecology: The Metaethics of Radical Feminism*. Boston: Beacon Press, 1978.
    See chapter 7 on "American Gynecology: Gynocide by the Holy Ghosts of Medicine and Therapy."

Dworkin, Andrea. *Right Wing Women*. New York: Perigee Books, 1983.
    See chapter 5 on "The Coming Gynocide," in which the author discusses the history and future of the control of women's rights and abilities, with an emphasis on the spirituality of women. She uses the analogies of a brothel model and a farming model.

Edwards, Margot and Mary Waldorf. *Reclaiming Birth: History and Heroines of American Childbirth Reform*. Trumansburg, NY: The Crossing Press, 1984.
    See especially Chapter 4: "The Saga of Obstetrical Technology."
    Historical and political discussion of electronic fetal monitoring (EFM), OB drugs, cesarean sections, ultrasound, episiotomies, etc.

Gordon, Linda. *Woman's Body, Woman's Right: A Social History of Birth Control in America*. New York: Grossman, 1976.
    An historical and political survey of birth control and abortion and some of their effects on American women.

Hastings Center Report, Journal of the Institute of Society, Ethics, and the Life Sciences, 360 Broadway, Hastings-on-Hudson, NY 10706.

Holmes, Helen B., Betty B. Hoskins and Michael Gross, eds. *Birth Control and Controlling Birth: Women-Centered Perspectives*. New Jersey: Humana Press, 1980.
    From the Conference on Ethical Issues in Reproductive Technology: Analysis by Women (EIRTAW), June 1979, Hampshire College, Amherst, MA.
    Workshop to identify ethical issues, determine which values have been considered, discover alternative values, and recom-

mend new approaches for determining policy. First of two volumes.

See especially Helen Holmes' introduction: "Reproductive Technologies: The Birth of a Woman-Centered Analysis" and the section on "Childbirth Technologies."

Holmes, Helen B., Betty B. Hoskins and Michael Gross, eds. *The Custom-Made Child: Women-Centered Perspectives*. New Jersey: Humana Press, 1981.

Second volume from the EIRTAW conference.

See especially "Prenatal Diagnosis" by Mary G. Ampola, "Technical Aspects of Sex Preselection" by Roberta Steinbacher, and the section on "Manipulative Reproductive Technologies."

Hubbard, Ruth, Mary Sue Henifin, and Barbara Fried, eds. *Biological Woman — The Convenient Myth: A Collection of Feminist Essays and a Comprehensive Bibliography*. Cambridge, MA: Schenkman Publishing Company, 1982.

See chapter by Jeanne M. Stellman and Mary Sue Henifin on employment discrimination and reproductive hazards in the workplace, chapter by Helen Rodriguez-Trias on sterilization abuse, and the bibliography.

Lappe, Marc. *Broken Code, The Exploitation of DNA*. San Francisco: Sierra Club Books, 1984.

See section entitled, "Recombinant DNA: Prospects for Health."

Lappe, Marc. *Genetic Politics: The Limits of Biological Control*. New York: Simon and Schuster, 1979.

McCormick, Richard. *How Brave a New World? Dilemmas in Bioethics*. Garden City, NY: Doubleday, 1981.

O'Brien, Mary. *The Politics of Reproduction*. Boston: Routledge and Kegan Paul, 1981.

Feminist political theory.

Rakusen, Jill and Nick Davidson. *Out of Our Hands: What Technology Does to Pregnancy*. London: Pan Books, 1982.

Reidy, Maurice, ed. *Ethical Issues in Reproductive Medicine*. Dublin: Gill and MacMillian, 1982.

Roberts, Helen, ed. *Women, Health and Reproduction*. Boston: Routledge and Kegan Paul, 1981.
    Discusses the gap between legitimated knowledge and personal experience, male control of childbirth, women's lack of access to health-related information, and alternative strategies, including abortion clinics and women's health clinics.
    See especially "Sex predetermination, artificial insemination and the maintenance of male-dominated culture" by Jalna Hanmer, pp. 163-190.

Sayers, Janet. *Biological Politics: Feminist and Anti-Feminist Perspectives*. London: Tavistock, 1982.

Singer, Peter and Deane Wells. *The Reproductive Revolution — New Ways of Making Babies*. New York: Oxford University Press, 1984.

Singer, Peter, and W. A. W. Walters, eds. *Test-Tube Babies: A Guide to Moral Questions, Present Techniques and Future Possibilities*. New York: Oxford University Press, 1982.

WomenWise: The New Hampshire Feminist Health Center Quarterly, 7(4), Winter 1984, p. 9.
    Available for $2.00 from The New Hampshire Feminist Health Center, 38 South Main Street, Concord, NH 03301/ (603) 225-2739 or 232 Court Street, Portsmouth, NH 03801/ (603) 436-7588.
    This entire issues focuses on reproductive technologies, including alpha-fetoprotein testing, cell fusion and parthenogenesis, and the issue of "choice" and disabilities.

B. Articles

Achilles, Rona. "Procreation in a New Age." *Healthsharing*, 10-14.
    A chilling comparison between science fiction and "science fact" in the area of reproductive technology. Interviews with medical researchers are interspersed with explanations of and documentaries on IVF, ultrasound, and other reproductive technologies.

Aral, Sevgi C. and Willard Cates. "The Increasing Concern with Infertility, Why Now?" *JAMA, 250*(17), 1983.

Arditti, Rita. "Scrutinizing New Reproductive Technologies." *Sojourner*, May 1985, 18-19.

Baruch, Elaine Hoffman and Amadeo F. D'Adamo, Jr. "Resetting the Biological Clock: Women and the New Reproductive Technologies." *Dissent*, Summer 1985, 273-276.

Bell, Susan et al. "Reclaiming Reproductive Control: A Feminist Approach to Fertility Consciousness." *Science for the People*, 12, 1980, 6-9, 30-35.

Brodribb, Somer. "Reproductive Technologies, Masculine Dominance, and the Canadian State." Occasional papers in Social Policy Analysis, Ontario Institute for Studies in Education (Toronto, Ontario), 1984.

Bunkle, Phillida, "Manufacturing Motherhood." *Broadsheet* (New Zealand), April 1984, 12-15, 23.

Cameron, Debbie, Elizabeth Agnes, Kathryn Eldith, and Maree Gladwin. "Reproductive Wrongs: Male Power and the New Reproductive Technologies." Manchester, UK: Amazon Press, 1984.
    Available from Sisterwrite, 190 Upper Street, London NI.
    This booklet, published by FINNRET, explains the technologies and recommends that women fight back against the

woman-hating and male violence which the authors believe they represent.

Corea, Gena. "Ethical Issues In Human Reproductive Technology: Analysis by Women." Somerville, 1979.
    Available from Boston Women's Health Book Collective, 47 Nichols Ave., Watertown, MA 02172.

Corea, Gena. "Unnatural Selection: The Menace of High-Tech Motherhood." *The Progressive*, January 1986, 22-24.

Courtney, Terry, et al. "Ethical Issues in Reproductive Technology: An Analysis by Women — Almost." *Off Our Backs*, 9, December 1979.

D'Adamo, Amadeo F. Jr. and Elaine Hoffman Baruch. "Whither the Womb? Myths, Machines and Mothers." *Frontiers: A Journal of Women's Studies* ix, no. 1, 1986, 72-79.

DeStefano, Thea and Helen Bequaert Holmes. "Human Genetic Manipulations: How Many Sides to the Coin?" *GeneWATCH*, 1(3 & 4), 3-6.

Duelli Klein, Renate, Gena Corea and Ruth Hubbard. "German Women Say NO to Gene and Reproductive Technology: Reflections on a Conference in Bonn, West Germany, April 19-21, 1985." "Feminist Forum" in *Women's Studies Int. Forum*, 8(3), 1985, pp. i-vi.
    ". . . a meeting *against* the technologies — not a pluralistic discussion on its supposed advantages and disadvantages for women." A denouncement, from a feminist viewpoint, of both gene and reproductive technologies.

The Economist. "Science and Technology: The Birthpangs of a New Science." July 14, 1984, 79-83.

Finkelstein, J. and P. Clough. "Foetal Politics and the Birth of an Industry." *Women's Studies International Forum*, 6(4), 1983, 395-400.

Gaill, Francoise, "Biologie et Feminisme." *CRIF Bulletin*, Centre de Recherches, de Reflexion et d'Information Feministes, Bulletin No. 8, Ete 1985.
In French.
A sociobiological critique, from the feminist perspective introduced by Simone de Beauvoir in *The Second Sex*, of reproduction and reproductive technologies. Gaill discusses reproduction as an action and a choice, despite biological constraints, and the dissociation of biological and social parenthood created by reproductive technologies.

Gorovitz, Samuel. "Obstetrical Intervention and Technology in the 1980's—The Ethical Issues." *Women and Health*, 7, Fall and Winter 1982, 1-7.

Hubbard, Ruth. "The Fetus as Patient." *Ms.*, 11(4), October 1982, 28-29.

Hubbard, Ruth and Mary Sue Henifin. "Genetic Screening of Prospective Parents and of Workers: Some Scientific and Social Issues." In: *Biomedical Ethics Review: 1984*. Edited by James M. Humber and Robert F. Almedar. Clifton, NJ: Humana Press, 1984, pp. 73-120.

Katz Rothman, Barbara. "How Science is Redefining Parenthood." *Ms.* July/August 1982.

Lappe, Marc. "Recombinant DNA: Prospects for Health." *GeneWATCH*, 1(5 & 6), 1, 16.
Also in: Marc Lappe. *Broken Code, The Exploitation of DNA*. San Francisco: Sierra Club Books, 1984.

Law, Sylvia. "Embryos and Ethics." *Family Planning Perspectives*, 17(3), 1985.

Lynn, Suzanne M. "Technology and Reproductive Rights: How Advances in Technology Can be Used to Limit Women's Reproductive Rights." *Reproductive Rights Symposium: Women's Rights Law Reporter*, 7(3), 1982.

Mies, Maria. "Why do we need all this? A Call Against Genetic Engineering and Reproductive Technology." *Women's Studies International Forum*, 8(6), July 1985, 553-560.

Minden, Shelley. "Genetic Engineering and Human Embryos." *Science for the People*, 17(3), 1985.

Minden, Shelley. "Patriarchal Designs: The Genetic Engineering of Human Embryos." *Women's Studies International Forum*, 8(6), July 1985, 561-566.

Rowland, Robyn, "A Child at ANY Price? An overview of issues in the use of the new reproductive technologies, and the threat to women." *Women's Studies International Forum*, 8(6), July 1985, 539-546.

Shaw, Evelyn and Joan Darling. "Maternalism – the Fathering of a Myth." *New Scientist*, February 14, 1985, 10-13.
    Laboratory experiments with animals yield evidence that males are as capable of '"maternal" behavior as females.

Singer, Peter. "Technology and Procreation: How Far Should We Go?" *Technology Review*, February/March 1985, 22-30.

Young, I. D. "Ethical Dilemmas in Clinical Genetics." *Journal of Medical Ethics*, 10, June 1984, 73-76.

II. LAW AND POLICY CONSIDERATIONS

Bowes, W. A. and D. Selgestad. "Fetal versus Maternal Rights: Medical and Legal Prospectives." *Obstetrics and Gynecology*, 58, August 1981, 209-214.

Engelhardt, H. T. "Current Controversies in Obstetrics: Wrongful Life and Forced Fetal Surgical Procedures." *American Journal of Obstetrics and Gynecology*, 151, 1 February 1985, 313-317.

Gallagher, Janet. "Fetal Personhood and Women's Policy," in Virginia Sapiro, ed. *Biology and Women's Policy*, Sage Yearbooks in Women's Policy Studies, Vol. 10. Beverly Hills: Sage Publications, 1985.

Gallagher, Janet. "The Fetus and the Law—Whose Life Is It Anyway?" *Ms.*, September 1984, 62-66, 134-135.

Hitchens, Donna. *Lesbians Choosing Motherhood: Legal Issues in Donor Insemination*. 1984 edition.
     Available for $5.00 from the Lesbian Rights Project, 1370 Mission Street, 4th Floor, San Francisco, CA 94103.

Hubbard, Ruth. "'Fetal Rights' and the New Eugenics." *Science for the People*, 16(2), March/April 1984, 7-9, 27-29.

Hubbard, Ruth. "Legal and Policy Implications of Recent Advances in Prenatal Diagnosis and Fetal Therapy," in *Reproductive Rights Symposium: Women's Rights Law Reporter*, 7(3), 1982.

King, Patricia. "The Juridicial Status of the Fetus: A Proposal for Legal Protection of the Unborn," *Michigan Law Review*, 77, 1979, 1647.

Milunsky, Aubrey and George Annas. *Genetics and The Law II*. New York: Plenum Press, 1980.

Milunsky, Aubrey and George Annas. *Genetics and the Law III*. New York: Plenum Press, 1985.

Ontario Law Reform Commission. *Report on Human Artificial Reproduction and Related Matters*. Ontario: Ministry of the Attorney General, 1985.

Reproductive Rights Law Reporter, 1524 Crescent Place, NW, Room 310, Washington, DC 20009.

Reproductive Rights National Network Bulletin, 17 Murray Street, 5th Floor, New York, NY 10007.

Safillos-Rothschild, C. *Women's Economic Autonomy and Fertility in the Third World*. WID Working Paper No. 13.

Available for $3.00 from: Women and International Development, Joint Harvard/MIT Group, Harvard Institute for International Development, 1737 Cambridge Street, Cambridge, MA 02138 (617) 495-4249.

Shaw, M. W. "Conditional Prospective Rights of the Fetus," *Journal of Legal Medicine*, 5, March 1984, 63.

III. INDIVIDUAL TECHNOLOGIES

A. Fetal Testing and Related Issues

Abortion Law Reform Association Newsletter/A Woman's Right to Choose Campaign. Available from: ALRA, 88A Islington High Street, London NI 8 EG England.

Andreano, R. L. and D. W. McCollum. "A Benefit-Cost Analysis of Amnio-Centesis." *Social Biology*, 30, Winter 1983, 347-373.
     An economic analysis of the use of amniocentesis for detecting and "avoiding" Down syndrome births.

Asch, Adrienne and Michell Fine. "Shared Dreams: A Left Perspective on Disability Rights and Reproductive Rights." *Radical America*, 18(4), July-August 1984.
     The authors discuss the biases against people with disabilities inherent in arguments about abortion of disabled fetuses and non-treatment of disabled infants, as well as their interpretation of the importance of the distinction between fetus and infant.

Blatt, Robin. "Prenatal Screening Test." *GeneWATCH*, 1(2), 1984.

Butler, Edith. "What Do We Know About Ultrasound?" *WomenWise: The New Hampshire Feminist Health Center Quarterly*, 7(4), Winter 1984, p. 9.
     Available for $2.00 from The New Hampshire Feminist Health Center, 38 South Main Street, Concord, NH 03301/

(603) 225-2739 or 232 Court Street, Portsmouth, NH 03801/ (603) 436-7588.
This entire issue focuses on reproductive technologies, including alpha-fetoprotein testing, cell fusion and parthenogenesis, and the issue of "choice" and disabilities.

English, Deirdre. "The War Against Choice: Inside the Antiabortion Movement." *Mother Jones*, 62, February/March 1981, 16-26.

Fineberg, K. S. and J. D. Peters. "Amniocentesis in Medicine and Law: Practice Standards and Legal Ramifications." *Trial*, 20, Fall 1984, 54-59.

Fletcher, J. C. "Ethical Issues in Genetic Screening and Antenatal Diagnosis." *Clinical Obstetrics and Gynecology*, 24, December 1981, 1151-1168.

Gilroy, F. and R. Steinbacher, eds. "Preselection of Child Sex: Technological Utilization and Feminism." *Psychological Reports*, 53, October 1983, 671-676.

Hanmer, Jalna. "Sex Predetermination, Artificial Insemination, and the Maintenance of Male-Dominated Culture," in Helen Roberts, ed. *Women, Health and Reproduction*. London: RKP, 1981.

Henry, Alice. "Selective Abortion—Thoughts from Several Countries." *Off Our Backs*, November 1984, 13-14.

Hubbard, Ruth. "Caring for Baby Doe." *Ms.*, 12(11), May 1984, 84-88, 165.

Hubbard, Ruth, "Prenatal Diagnosis and Eugenic Ideology." *Women's Studies International Forum*, 8(6), July 1985, 561-566.

Hubbard, Ruth. "Prenatal Diagnosis and Fetal Therapy: Legal and Policy Implications." *Women's Rights Law Reporter*, 7(3), Spring 1982.

Huether, C. A. "Projection of Down's Syndrome Births in the United States 1979-2000, and the Potential Effects of Prenatal Diagnosis." *American Journal of Public Health*, 73, October 1983, 1186-1189.

    Proposes amniocentesis for pregnant women over age 32 or 33 in order to reduce the number of children born with Down Syndrome.

Kaiser, I. H. "Amniocentesis." *Women and Health*, 7, Fall and Winter 1982, 29-38.

Kolata, Gina. "Beyond Amniocentesis: New Techniques in Fetal Testing." *Ms.*, December 1983, 91-94.

    A summary of techniques for alpha fetoprotein (AFP) screening, ultrasound, amniocentesis and chorionic villus biopsy, and a discussion of birth defects. Kolata cautions women to become informed about the necessity and risks of such techniques.

Milunsky, Aubrey. *The Prenatal Diagnosis of Hereditary Disorders*. Springfield, IL: Thomas, 1973.

Nielsen, C. C. "An Encounter with Modern Medical Technology: Women's Experiences with Amniocentesis." *Women and Health*, 6, Spring and Summer 1981, 109-129.

Orkin, Stuart H. "Genetic Diagnosis of the Fetus." *Nature*, 296, 1982, 202-3.

Patychuck, Dianne. "Ultrasound: The First Wave." *Healthsharing*, Fall 1985, 25-28.

Perry, T. B. et al. "Chorionic Villi Sampling: Clinical Experience, Immediate Complications, and Patient Attitudes." *American Journal of Obstetrics and Gynecology*, 251, 15 January 1985, 161-166.

Petchesky, Rosalind. *Abortion and Women's Choice*. New York: Longman, 1984.

President's Commission for the Study of Ethical Problems in Medicine and Biomedical and Behavioral Research. *Screening and*

Counseling for Genetic Conditions. Superintendant of Documents, U.S. Government Printing Office, Washington, DC 20402. 1983.

Rapp, Rayna. "The Ethics of Choice: After My Amniocentesis, Mike and I Faced the Toughest Decision of Our Lives." *Ms.*, April 1984, 97.
    A personal account of the decision-making process after amniocentesis and the effects on one couple's decision.

Rayburn, W. F. "Clinical Implications from Monitoring Fetal Activity." *American Journal of Obstetrics and Gynecology*, 144, 15 December 1982, 967-980.

Singer, Peter and Helga Kuhse. "The Future of Baby Doe." *The New York Review*, March 1, 1984, 17-22.

Steinbacher, Roberta. "Sex Pre-selection: From Here to Fraternity," in Carol Gould, ed., *Beyond Domination: New Perspectives on Women and Philosophy*. Totowa, NJ: Littlefield and Adams, 1983.

Stinson, Robert and Peggy Stinson. *The Long Dying of Baby Andrew*. Boston: Little, Brown, 1983.
    A personal account of one couple's struggle upon learning, through amniocentesis, that the woman was carrying a fetus which would be born with a serious genetic defect.

Volodkevich, H. and C. A. Huether. "Causes of Low Utilization of Amniocentesis by Women of Advanced Maternal Age." *Social Biology*, 28, Fall-Winter 1981, 176-186.
    Concludes that many women of advanced maternal age, if adequately "counseled" by their doctors, would choose to undergo amniocentesis and to abort Down Syndrome fetuses.

Williamson, Nancy. *Sons or Daughters: A Cross-Cultural Survey of Parental Preferences*. Russell Sage, New York: Sage Library of Social Research, 1976.

B. Technologies Affecting Conception

1. *In Vitro* Fertilization

Corea, Genoveffa and Susan Ince. "IVF a Game for Losers at Half of US Clinics." *Medical Tribune*, International Medical News Weekly, 26(19), July 3, 1985.
> An analysis of the true success and failure rates of IVF clinics and the use of misleading statistics by many of them.

Crowe, Christine, "Women Want It: In-Vitro Fertilization and Women's Motivations for Participation." *Women's Studies International Forum*, 8(6), July 1985, 547-552.

Freeman, E. W., et al. "Psychological Evaluation and Support in a Program of *In Vitro* Fertilization and Embryo Transfer." *Fertility and Sterility*, 43, January 1985, 48-53.

Gold, Michael. "The Baby Makers." *Science 85*, April 1985, 26-38.
> Interviews and information about Howard and Georgeanna Jones' IVF clinic at Eastern Virginia Medical School in Norfolk — the nation's most successful IVF clinic.

Grobstein, Clifford. *From Chance to Purpose: An Appraisal of External Human Fertilization*. Reading, MA: Addison-Wesley Publishing Company, 1981.
> A technological introduction to IVF with a relatively thorough analysis of ethical issues relating to the fetus, but the rights of the mother are addressed only superficially, if at all.

Iglesias, T. "*In Vitro* Fertilization: The Major Issues." *Journal of Medical Ethics*, 10, March 1984, 38-44.

Kirby, M. D. "Bioethics of IVF — The State of the Debate." *Journal of Medical Ethics*, *10*, March 1984, 45-48.

Olson, Maleia and Nancy J. Alexander. *In-Vitro Fertilization and Embryo Transfer*. Oregon: Oregon Health Sciences University, 1984.

Singer, P. and D. Wells. *"In Vitro* Fertilization: The Major Issues."* Journal of Medical Ethics*, 9, December 1983, 192-195.

Tiefel, Hans O. "Human *In Vitro* Fertilization: A Conservative View." *JAMA*, 247(23), 18 June 1982, 3235-3242.
    Focuses on moral rights of embryo. Makes some reference to parents, society.

Turner, Jill. *In Vitro Fertilization and Embryo Transfer—Just the Tip of the Iceberg*. Unpubl. Dissertation, Interdisciplinary Human Studies, University of Bradford, 1984.

Zaner, R. M. "A Criticism of Moral Conservatism's View of *In Vitro* Fertilization and Embryo Transfer." *Perspectives in Biology and Medicine*, 27, Winter 1984, 200-212.
    Response to Tiefel's paper (see above). Also focuses on fetus.

2. Artificial Insemination

Artificial Insemination Packet. Lesbian Mother National Defense Fund, PO Box 21567, Seattle, WA 98111. 1981. $3.00.
    A self-help guide to the medical and legal aspects of artificial insemination by donor.

Davis, J. H. and D. W. Brown. "Artificial Insemination by Donor and the Use of Surrogate Mothers—Social and Psychological Impact." *The Western Journal of Medicine*, 141, July 1984, 127-131.

Leiblum, S. R. and C. Barbrack. "Artificial Insemination by Donor: Survey of Attitudes and Knowledge in Medical Students and Infertile Couples." *The Journal of Biosocial Science*, 15, April 1983, 165-172.

Pizer, H. F., PAC, and S. Robinson, MD. *Having a Baby Without a Man: A Woman's Guide to Alternative Insemination*. New York: Simon and Schuster, 1985.

Self-Insemination.
>   Available from the Feminist Self-Insemination Group, PO
>   Box 3, 190 Upper Street, London NI, United Kingdom. 1980.

C. Sterilization and Contraception

CARASA
Committee for Abortion Rights and Against Sterilization Abuse
17 Murray Street, 5th Floor, New York, NY 10007

Committee for Abortion Rights and Against Sterilization Abuse.
Women Under Attack: Abortion, Sterilization Abuse, and Reproductive Freedom. New York: CARASA, 1979.

Curlin, P., and B. Brown. *Fertility and Choice: Increasing Women's Choices Through Women-Managed Service Delivery Programs.* WID Working Paper No. 9.
>   Available for $3.00 from: Women and International Development, Joint Harvard/MIT Group, Harvard Institute for International Development, 1737 Cambridge Street, Cambridge, MA 02138 (617) 495-4249.

Gulati, L. *Fertility and Choice in Kerala: Some Insights.* WID Working Paper No. 12.
>   Available for $3.00 from: Women and International Development, Joint Harvard/MIT Group, Harvard Institute for International Development, 1737 Cambridge Street, Cambridge, MA 02138 (617) 495-4249.

Kaufman, J. *Fertility and Choice for Women in China.* WID Working Paper No. 11.
>   Available for $3.00 from: Women and International Development, Joint Harvard/MIT Group, Harvard Institute for International Development, 1737 Cambridge Street, Cambridge, MA 02138 (617) 495-4249.

Lukas, A., and J. Kulig. *Bridging the Gap: Birth Practices, Birth Control, and Sexuality Among Cambodian and Vietnamese Refugee Women.* WID Working Paper No. 10.

Available for $3.00 from: Women and International Development, Joint Harvard/MIT Group, Harvard Institute for International Development, 1737 Cambridge Street, Cambridge MA 02138 (617) 495-4249.

Safilios-Rothschild, C. *Women's Economic Autonomy and Fertility in the Third World*. WID Working Paper No. 13.
Available for $3.00 from: Women and International Development, Joint Harvard/MIT Group, Harvard Institute for International Development, 1737 Cambridge Street, Cambridge, MA 02138 (617) 495-4249.

Smith, G. L. "Comparative Risks and Costs of Male and Female Sterilization. *American Journal of Public Health*, 75, April 1975, p. 370.

Veevers, J. E. "Differential Childlessness by Color: A Further Examination." *Social Biology*, 29, Spring/Summer 1982, 180-186.

Welch, C. E. "The Regulation of American Fertility: Facts and Misconceptions." *International Journal of Women's Studies*, 7, 1984, 273-281.

IV. FURTHER REFERENCES

A. Periodicals

GeneWATCH, Bulletin of the Committee for Responsible Genetics, 5 Doane Street, 4th Floor, Boston, MA 02109.

Hastings Center Report, Journal of the Institute of Society, Ethics, and the Life Sciences, 360 Broadway, Hastings-on-Hudson, NY 10706.

Healthright. 41 Union Square, Room 206-209, New York, NY 10003.

Healthsharing: A Canadian Women's Health Quarterly, 101 Niagara Street, Suite 200A, Toronto, Ontario M5V 1C3.

Maternal Health News. Available from: Maternal Health Society, Box 46563, Station G, Vancouver VGR 4G8, Canada.

Mothering: A Quarterly by Mothering Publications, Inc., PO Box 2208, Albuquerque, NM 87103.

National Women's Health Network News. 224 Seventh Street SE, Washington, DC 20003.

Reproductive Rights Law Reporter, 1624 Crescent Place, NW, Room 310, Washington, DC 20009.

Reproductive Rights National Network Bulletin, 17 Murray Street, 5th Floor, New York, NY 10097.

B. Organizations

Boston Women's Health Book Collective
47 Nickols Avenue
Watertown, MA 02172

CARASA
Committee for Abortion Rights and Against Sterilization Abuse
17 Murray Street, 5th Floor
New York, NY 10007

Committee to Defend Reproductive Rights
2845 24th Street
San Francisco, CA 94110
(415) 826-4401

Committee for Responsible Genetics
Women and Reproductive Technology Project
186A South Street
Boston, MA 02111
(617) 423-0650

FINRRAGE
Feminist International Network of Resistance to Reproductive and Genetic Engineering
(Formerly FINNRET: Feminist International Network on the New Reproductive Technologies)

U.S. Contact: FINNRET
Janice Raymond
Women's Studies
University of Massachusetts
Amherst, MA 01003

FINRRAGE
Gena Corea
PO Box 751
Winchester, MA 01890

International: FINRRAGE
Renate Duelli Klein
PO Box 583
London NW3 IRQ
England

Lesbians Choosing Children Network
46 Pleasant Street
Cambridge, MA 02139
(617) 354-8807

National Women's Health Network
224 Seventh Street SE
Washington, DC 20003
(202) 543-9222

R₂N₂
Reproductive Rights National Network
17 Murray Street, 5th floor
New York, NY 10007
(212) 267-8891

C. Bibliographies

Bibliography of Society, Ethics and the Life Sciences. Hastings-on-the-Hudson: Institute of Society, Ethics and the Life Sciences, 1970-1980.
See section on "Genetics, Fertilization, and Birth."

Cowan, Belita. *Women's Health Care: Resources, Writings, Bibliographies*. Ann Arbor: Anshen, 1977.

A good bibliography of women's health, but not recent enough to include much information about the new reproductive technologies.

Een, J. D., and M. B. Rosenberg-Dishman (compilers). *Women and Society:* Citations 3601-6000: An Annotated Bibliography. Beverly Hills: Sage Publication, 1978.
See section on women in medicine and health.

The Hastings Center's Bibliography of Ethics, Biomedicine and Professional Responsibility. University Publications of America, 1984.

Hubbard, Ruth, Mary Sue Henifin, and Barbara Fried, eds. *Biological Women – The Convenient Myth*: A Collection of Feminist Essays and a Comprehensive Bibliography. Cambridge, MA: Schenkman Publishing Company, 1982.

Johnsen, A. R., et al. "The Ethics of Medicine: An Annotated Bibliography of Recent Literature." *Annals of Internal Medicine*, 92, 1980, 136- .

Meyer, S. I. "Bibliography" [Women and Health Care]. *Women & Health*, 7, 1982, 67-75.

Reich W. T. (ed). *Encyclopedia of Bioethics*, Vol. 4 & 5. New York: The Free Press, 1978.
See especially the following sections:
"Reproductive Technologies," vol. 4, pp. 1439-1470.
"Genetic Diagnosis and Counseling," vol. 5, pp. 555-566.
"Genetic Screening," vol. 5, pp. 567-572.
"Prenatal Diagnosis," vol. 5, pp. 1332-1346.

"Reproductive Rights." In: *Sourcebook: Building Bridges, Not Walls*. New York: 16th National Conference on Women and the Law, 1985, 96-100.

Selected Bibliography on New Reproductive Technologies. Boston: Women and Reproductive Technology Project of the Committee for Responsible Genetics, 1985.

Available from the Committee for Responsible Genetics, 186A South Street, Boston, MA 02111.

Sutterley, D., and E. Schachne (compilers). *Health Care, Medical Ethics, and Reproductive Issues: A Working Bibliography, 1977-1985*. Princeton University: Program in Women's Studies, 1985.
Available from the Program in Women's Studies, 218 Palmer Hall, Princeton University, Princeton NJ 08544.

Women and Women's Rights: A Medical, Psychological and International Subject Survey with Research Index and Bibliography. Washington, DC: ABBE Publishers Association of Washington, DC, 1984.